Thriving in Mental Health Nursing

Laura Duncan

*Senior Lecturer at The University of Chester,
Primary Care Network Lead at Cheshire and
Wirral Partnership NHS Foundation Trust,
Nursing and Midwifery Council Registered
Nurse in Mental Health,
Teaching Fellow with The Higher Education Academy*

WILEY Blackwell

This edition first published 2025
© 2025 John Wiley & Sons Ltd

All rights reserved, including rights for text and data mining and training of artificial technologies or similar technologies. No part of this publication may be reproduced, stored in a retrieval system, or transmitted, in any form or by any means, electronic, mechanical, photocopying, recording or otherwise, except as permitted by law. Advice on how to obtain permission to reuse material from this title is available at http://www.wiley.com/go/permissions.

The right of Laura Duncan to be identified as the author of this work has been asserted in accordance with law.

Registered Offices
John Wiley & Sons, Inc., 111 River Street, Hoboken, NJ 07030, USA
John Wiley & Sons Ltd, New Era House, 8 Oldlands Way, Bognor Regis, West Sussex, PO22 9NQ, UK

For details of our global editorial offices, customer services, and more information about Wiley products visit us at www.wiley.com.

Wiley also publishes its books in a variety of electronic formats and by print-on-demand. Some content that appears in standard print versions of this book may not be available in other formats.

Trademarks: Wiley and the Wiley logo are trademarks or registered trademarks of John Wiley & Sons, Inc. and/or its affiliates in the United States and other countries and may not be used without written permission. All other trademarks are the property of their respective owners. John Wiley & Sons, Inc. is not associated with any product or vendor mentioned in this book.

Limit of Liability/Disclaimer of Warranty
The contents of this work are intended to further general scientific research, understanding, and discussion only and are not intended and should not be relied upon as recommending or promoting scientific method, diagnosis, or treatment by physicians for any particular patient. In view of ongoing research, equipment modifications, changes in governmental regulations, and the constant flow of information relating to the use of medicines, equipment, and devices, the reader is urged to review and evaluate the information provided in the package insert or instructions for each medicine, equipment, or device for, among other things, any changes in the instructions or indication of usage and for added warnings and precautions. While the publisher and authors have used their best efforts in preparing this work, they make no representations or warranties with respect to the accuracy or completeness of the contents of this work and specifically disclaim all warranties, including without limitation any implied warranties of merchantability or fitness for a particular purpose. No warranty may be created or extended by sales representatives, written sales materials or promotional statements for this work. This work is sold with the understanding that the publisher is not engaged in rendering professional services. The advice and strategies contained herein may not be suitable for your situation. You should consult with a specialist where appropriate. The fact that an organization, website, or product is referred to in this work as a citation and/or potential source of further information does not mean that the publisher and authors endorse the information or services the organization, website, or product may provide or recommendations it may make. Further, readers should be aware that websites listed in this work may have changed or disappeared between when this work was written and when it is read. Neither the publisher nor authors shall be liable for any loss of profit or any other commercial damages, including but not limited to special, incidental, consequential, or other damages.

Library of Congress Cataloging-in-Publication Data Applied for:

Paperback ISBN: 9781394202355

Cover Design: Wiley
Cover Image: © Shaumiaa Vector/Getty Images

Set in 10/12pt STIXTwoText by Straive, Pondicherry, India
Printed and bound by CPI Group (UK) Ltd, Croydon, CR0 4YY
C9781394202355_091224

This book is dedicated to all of the incredible mental health professionals that I have had the pleasure of working with throughout my career. Thank you to everyone for not only the incredible work you do but the support that you give every day.

To my husband Sam, thank you for all that you do to lift me up and encourage me. Without you, this book would not have been possible. To my friends and family, I'm sure you'll all be thrilled that it is finally complete! Thank you especially to my wonderful parents for your unwavering belief and unending support of me over the years.

Laura Duncan

CONTENTS

1 Introduction   1

2 Reflection   3
    Activity,   4
    Vignettes,   4
    Vignette,   7
    Activity,   8
    References,   9

3 Resilience   11
    Activity,   14
    Vignette,   15
    References,   17

4 Emotional Intelligence   19
    Activity,   20
    Case Study,   21
    References,   23

5 Listening and Communication Skills   25
    Activity,   27
    Case Study,   28
    References,   31

6 Working with Trauma 33
Activities, 36
References, 40

7 Working with Risk 41
Activities, 43
   How to Approach Difficult Questions, 43
   What Happens When Risk Assessments Go Wrong and How Do We Manage Our Feelings?, 46
References, 47

8 Diversity and Inclusivity 49
Activity, 56
References, 58

9 Managing Therapeutic Relationships 61
Activities, 63
   Developing a Therapeutic Relationship, 63
   Maintaining a Therapeutic Relationship, 65
   Ending a Therapeutic Relationship, 66
References, 67

10 Managing Complexity 69
Activity, 71
Vignette, 72
References, 73

11 Conflict 75
Activity, 76
Case Study, 78
Activity, 79
Vignette, 80
References, 81

Contents   ix

12 Compassion   83

Activity, 85
Activity, 86
Vignettes, 86
References, 88

13 Maintaining Hope   89

Vignette 1, 90
Vignette 2, 91
Activity, 93
References, 93

14 Self-Care and Well-being   95

Activities, 97
References, 99

15 Burnout   101

Activity, 102
Case Study, 105
References, 107

16 Stigma and Discrimination   109

Public Stigma Case Study, 110
Structural Stigma Case Study, 110
Courtesy Stigma, 110
Provider-Based Stigma, 111
Self-Stigma Case Study, 111
  Mind Your Language!, 115
  Be Kind, Always, 118
  Challenge Others, 118
References, 118

17 Ethical Practice 121

    Activity, 123
    Case Study, 125
    Outcome, 126
    References, 127

18 Working in Teams 129

    Activity, 129
    Activity, 130
    Integrating Case Study, 131
    Compromising Case Study, 132
    Dominating Case Study, 132
    Avoiding Case Study, 133
    Obliging Case Study, 134
    References, 135

19 Leadership 137

    Case Studies, 140
    Activity, 144
    References, 145

20 Supervision Skills 147

    Activities, 150
      Reflective Activity, 150
    Case Studies, 150
      Case Study 1, 150
      Case Study 2, 151
    References, 152

21 Professional Development 153

    Activity, 154
    References, 158

22 Social Determinants of Health Chapter   159

Agriculture and Food Production Case Study,   161
Education Case Study,   161
Work Environment Case Study,   162
Unemployment Case Study,   162
Water and Sanitation Case Study,   163
Healthcare Services Case Study,   163
Housing Case Study,   164
Social Prescribing Case Study,   166
References,   167

23 The Biopsychosocial Model   169

Schizophrenia Case Study,   170
Biological,   171
Psychological,   172
Social,   172
References,   173

24 The Stress Vulnerability Model   175

Case Study,   177
References,   178

25 Accessing Support   181

Activity,   182
References,   184

26 Final Thoughts   185

INDEX   **187**

CHAPTER 1

Introduction

Mental health nursing is an incredible profession that I have been proud to have been part of throughout my career. It provides the opportunity to help people in a very real way and that is incredibly rewarding. It is also a very challenging role and this is for many reasons. As Mental Health professionals, we work with individuals who are in distress and experiencing the worst moments of their lives, and this can take a significant toll on us over time. We witness things that no other professional group outside of health and social care usually would, and that is just a standard day at the office. Many books focus on how to understand and support clients better, and this is a part of this text as well, but the much bigger message is how to support ourselves and our teams.

One of the biggest issues facing mental health nurses currently is staffing levels, stress and burnout. The role has never been an easy one but additional pressures and demands have meant that nurses are leaving the profession in significant and terrifying numbers. If we are to protect the profession and clients, we must protect ourselves. Understanding how to manage burnout when we see it in ourselves, and in others, may mean that that individual is able to continue and thrive in the profession. Understanding that we are human and sometimes we need a break is the best way to protect ourselves from the terrible effects of burnout.

The core focus of this book is to help professionals have long, happy, successful and healthy careers. There is a strong focus on our own well-being and how to recognise the impact of specific issues, such as working with trauma, conflict and risk, as well as what to do about this if it impacts you negatively. It discusses how to recognise and improve key skillsets such as communication, reflection and resilience with a focus not only on being better able to support clients but also on increasing job satisfaction and well-being for ourselves as well. There will be consideration of how to understand and work effectively with clients across all needs and presentations with particular focus on key models such as The stress vulnerability model and the biopsychosocial model.

Thriving in Mental Health Nursing, First Edition. Laura Duncan.
© 2025 John Wiley & Sons Ltd. Published 2025 by John Wiley & Sons Ltd.

Chapter 1 Introduction

'You can't pour from an empty cup' is a phrase we hear frequently in nursing and we all know this to be true. We often say this to others when we know they are struggling but how much time do we spend thinking about how to refill our cup? Self-care is a key theme within this book, and we frequently overlook the importance of actually caring for ourselves as we spend so much of our time and energy caring for others. If we are to thrive as professionals, we need to proactively care for our own needs but also identify when we may need additional support.

In each chapter, there is a discussion of the key principles of each topic with activities, case studies and vignettes used to apply the theory to practice. The intent of this is to make it feel more 'real' and less like a purely theoretical or academic interpretation. The case studies and vignettes are all based on my own personal experiences in clinical practice so they will hopefully be realistic and 'true to life'. There are reflective activities throughout that are intended to help us to think about our own attitudes, thoughts and approaches in a considered way. Some of these may feel challenging to engage with but will hopefully help to build reflective skills in particular.

Mental health nursing is a unique, challenging and rewarding profession to be a part of. The one thing we can guarantee in this field is that you will never be bored! The variety of roles and the constant development and expansion of these roles means that Mental Health is an exciting and dynamic industry to work in. In comparison to general medicine, we are a new and emerging field. New understanding and developments are happening all the time, and if we reflect on where we were only 10 years ago, we can see how rapidly the profession is changing and adapting.

We spend our careers helping others to understand their thoughts, feelings and emotions. Hopefully, after reading this, we will understand our own and their impact better too. If we are to truly thrive as professionals, we must focus on the well-being of our clients, teams and ourselves.

CHAPTER 2

Reflection

Reflection as a concept is about looking at our thoughts, feelings and actions and evaluating them. It is about analysing our reactions, those of our team and the impact of these upon our clients. Reflection is about understanding what we did well, what we did not do well and how we could improve in the future. Becoming a reflective practitioner who is able to consider our own strengths and weaknesses with a view to continual improvement should be the goal of every registered nurse and healthcare professional.

Reflection is a core concept within nursing, and it is a key feature of any modern nursing programme. The emphasis on the importance of reflection is fairly recent, and many of us who trained more than 10 years ago will have first completed a written reflection for revalidation when that became a core aspect of the process (Nursing and Midwifery Council (NMC), n.d.), but without this being included in our training, many of us have struggled with formal reflections. My first reflections for revalidation under the NMC standards were deeply unreflective! Reading back now, I can see clearly that they are merely descriptions of a situation without any deeper understanding of them. I have shown these 'reflections' to students as a learning exercise and invited critique, the first comment is always 'they aren't very reflective'. Now, registered nurses must write reflective accounts every 3 years; they may have 'reflective practice' sessions within their clinical team or they may ask student nurses to write reflections after an incident or issue. This is all absolutely fine, of course, but what many don't recognise is that to be effective practitioners, we should always be reflecting.

Reflection is like any other skill, the more it is practised, the easier and more fluid it becomes. We can start with a theory-based model to support us through our initial reflections, but many will find this to be a tedious and time-consuming model with little new insight achieved. It is, however, essential to learn about the reflective models, similar to learning your scales when playing an instrument. Utilising a model such as Gibbs' reflective cycle (Gibbs and Andrew, 2001) and following the stages of

- Description of the event (what happened?)
- Feelings (what were you thinking and feeling when the event occurred?)
- Evaluation (what was good and bad about the situation and how it occurred?)

Thriving in Mental Health Nursing, First Edition. Laura Duncan.
© 2025 John Wiley & Sons Ltd. Published 2025 by John Wiley & Sons Ltd.

- Analysis (what else can you find about the situation?)
- Conclusion (what else could you have done?)
- Action plan (if it arose again, what would you do?)

This can help to build and develop our early reflective skills. Following the cycle of reflection in a structured and repeated way helps to develop and make it into our muscle memory, again, like learning scales! What many people do, however, is only reflect on the big situations, such as an assault or an error that has occurred, and where reflection is, of course, very helpful in these scenarios, we should also be reflecting on the everyday situations and things that have gone well. Sometimes, there may have been a difficult incident that has occurred, and the reflection from it is that actually, this couldn't have been prevented or handled in a different manner that would have changed the outcome. To become a truly 'reflective practitioner', we need to be reflecting almost all the time.

Activity

- Think about a scenario that you have been involved in recently that went better than expected.
- Follow Gibbs' reflective cycle steps (above) to analyse the incident.
- Focus mainly on your feelings, if you have used a single adjective such as 'it made me happy', try and dig into that a little deeper. Was it just happy, or were you 'proud' of your work? Were you 'hopeful' for the other person? Were you 'excited' about the outcome?
- Review what you wrote for the 'Evaluation' section. The task was to reflect on a positive scenario, is your evaluation more positive than negative? If not, have another think and try and identify more positives in the scenario.
- What was your action plan? 'I'd do it exactly the same again' is still an action plan; we don't have to find action points that aren't necessary if it has been a positive outcome. An action plan could be 'I'd approach the situation with more confidence next time because I know it has gone well before' and that would be accurate and effective.

Vignettes

In this chapter, I will use two vignettes to demonstrate the concepts being discussed. I will first explore a reflection utilising Gibbs' reflective model (Gibbs and Andrew, 2001), as I have tasked you with doing in the activity section. The second vignette will come later and explore more informal reflective principles.

- Description of the event
    - In my role as a lecturer, I support many students during their studies and journey to becoming a nurse. For some students, this journey is not straightforward, and they may need to take a break from their studies for a number of reasons. I recently met with one student who has been having a very difficult time in her personal life, and her mental health was ultimately not good. She was struggling with many things, her mood being very bad, and it was having a negative effect on her studies. I have been a lecturer for a long time and have

worked with several thousand students, many of whom have struggled during their programme and I can recognise that this is becoming an untenable situation for this particular student. She was struggling to an extent that she was going to start failing or missing assignments and practice placements. I can objectively see that taking a break from her studies to rest and recover will be more beneficial than struggling and possibly ending her studies because of failing assignments or her placements. We had a meeting, and after discussing all of the options and my concerns for her, she agreed to take a break from her studies and to seek help. She was very upset during our meeting, but we came to an agreement that this was the best way forward and that she can focus on her own well-being now so that she can return and complete the programme to achieve her dream of becoming a mental health nurse.

- Feelings
  - Going into the meeting, I was very nervous; I was worried there would be a negative outcome to the meeting, that I would cause further distress to the student, and that she could be in crisis if I did not handle this well. I was very conscious of listening to her thoughts and feelings throughout the meeting and being supportive of her when she was tearful and upset. I left the meeting feeling satisfied with the outcome and that this was the most supportive and positive action for her, but guilty that it had upset her. I was concerned for her well-being and was ruminating on whether I had done the right thing for several days to come.
- Evaluation
  - Overall, it was a positive outcome, and the student recognised that also. It was the right decision as she was not in a good place and could not focus on her studies; taking a few months to seek support, rest, and recover was the correct decision for her to be able to complete the programme successfully and achieve everything she wanted to in the future. I gave her space to be upset and to ask questions and supported her in reflecting on the situation herself to come to the conclusion that taking a break was the right decision. I didn't rush the meeting; we talked about support mechanisms and what to do if she was further distressed or in crisis, and she agreed that she would seek support. One reflective tool that had a particularly strong effect was asking her what advice she would give to one of her peers who was going through everything she was; after some thought, she responded 'to take a break'. I think that was a particularly strong realisation for her and supported her to recognise her clinical skills and knowledge.
- Analysis
  - This is a scenario I have been in many times and will likely be in again and so reflecting upon it is important. I think the meeting itself went as well as it could have done; I believe the student understood that I cared about their well-being and their future, and that is a really positive outcome from the situation. Recognising the student's knowledge and skills was important and hopefully, this was empowering for her. I was very conscious of being positive and future focussed on how she would feel better, return to her studies, and thrive as a mental health nurse, which I truly believe is the case, and I think that maintaining that hope for her when she maybe couldn't feel that herself at the moment was important.
- Conclusion
  - I found myself worrying after the meeting had occurred, whether I had done the right thing, said the right things, etc., but completing this reflection has helped me identify that this was always going to be a difficult conversation that would be emotional in nature. I demonstrated my commitment and care to her studies and achievements throughout. A separate reflection

to complete would be about whether, in the months preceding this, I had recognised that her mental health was deteriorating and if I could have intervened sooner to support her. I think my clinical skills in nursing were important as I was able to help her reflect, process her emotions with her and maintain hope for her.
- Action Plan
  - I will of course keep in contact with this student to support her, particularly when she returns to the programme, as that may be challenging for her. I will have more confidence in my skills in similar scenarios moving forward and will try and identify sooner when students may be struggling to try and put measures in to support them earlier.

As you can hopefully see from the reflection above, I focussed mainly on my thoughts and feelings. This can be very challenging, often because as mental health professionals, we can struggle to accept our own emotions and feelings are part of any interaction. It would have been emotionally easier to focus on the student's emotions within the reflection and they are, of course, important and acknowledged within the reflection; however, this is a reflection about me as the lecturer and professional in this scenario. The process behind the situation was very straightforward and something I have done several hundred times, so a functional focus would not have been particularly beneficial as the process is always the same and instructed by university policy. It is difficult to acknowledge my feelings in this scenario; however, this is an important aspect of processing these feelings as after completing the above reflection, I feel more confident that I acted appropriately, in a supportive manner, and ultimately handled the situation well. There are of course learning points, and a key action point would be trying to identify how to support students who may be struggling sooner, which, of course, is a significant challenge. Acknowledging that I had actually been ruminating on the situation – ultimately due to guilt of not identifying the seriousness of the situation sooner and causing further upset to the student – was something that I hadn't actually recognised until completing the reflection. It can be difficult to notice or recognise that we are having ongoing feelings or reactions to particular scenarios that have occurred. and sometimes these can present in different ways. When something is playing on my mind, as this scenario did, I find I can become snappy and irritable about small things but after reflection, can identify it is because of something else much bigger that I haven't been able to fully process and move forward from.

As we have explored above, Gibbs' reflective cycle (Gibbs and Andrew, 2001) can be very helpful as a formal reflective model, particularly when we need additional prompting to explore our thoughts and feelings in relation to a situation but there are other models of reflection that can also be very helpful. One such model is Driscoll's Model of Reflection (2007) in which there are just three stages:

- What? (Describe the situation/scenario. What exactly happened? What did you do? What did others do?)
- So what? (Why is it important? What happened, and how was it resolved? How did it make you feel?)
- Now what? (How do you move forward? Are there any further actions to take to resolve the situation? Do you need support or to escalate the situation? What have you learned? What could you do better to prepare yourself for similar situations in the future?)

Driscoll's (2007) model is possibly the simplest reflective model in terms of its structure and so becomes a frequently used and cited model. The simplicity of the model does not mean that the reflection it prompts from the clinician or practitioner is any less detailed or in-depth; however, the individual reflecting and utilising this model will need to challenge themselves more to reflect in an effective, detailed and in-depth manner.

Vignette

As discussed above, we will now explore more informal reflective principles, utilising Driscoll's (2007) model.

At the beginning of my career in mental health nursing, I worked in a psychiatric intensive care unit and then a triage assessment unit within the same mental health unit. I lived approximately a 30-minute walk from work, and I would normally get the bus to work but would always walk home from my shift. During my walk home, I would think about the shift that had just happened, and although I wasn't utilising Driscoll's (2007) model at the time (as I wasn't aware of it!), it could be argued that I was following the core principles.

During my walk home, I would think about what had happened during that shift (What?), had there been any incidents? Had there been any challenges? I would then think about my reactions to them (So what?); had I acted correctly? Had I responded quickly enough? Had I read the warning signs correctly? Had I followed the appropriate policy? Had I documented thoroughly enough? Then, I would think about what I would do differently on the next shift (Now what?); did I need to raise anything with my supervisor or ward manager? Did I need to ask for help in understanding something better? Do I need more training? Are there any improvements within the team I could identify?

I would allow myself to ruminate on all of these things throughout my walk home, including allowing myself to feel whatever emotion occurred. Did I feel unsupported? Was I angry at something that had happened? Had something upsetting or distressing happened? I would feel my feelings and think of what I needed to do next time I was on shift all the way home, and then I would close the door. I would close the door literally and metaphorically – and once I was at home, work was done – and it would not be allowed in. I was semi-cognisant of this approach and that I used the door as a way of maintaining my work–life balance, but that was pretty easy in that role. No work came home with me, I didn't need to check my emails when I wasn't on shift, and I couldn't in any way 'work from home' so that definitive boundary was very easy to maintain. What I didn't fully recognise or appreciate at the time was that I was informally reflecting all the way home and that having such a firm boundary and switching into 'home Laura' as soon as I was through the door was an incredibly healthy way of processing an emotionally difficult and demanding role.

Reflecting upon my informal reflection style at the earliest part of my career, I can recognise that without having the awareness of reflective models such as Gibbs' (Gibbs and Andrew, 2001) or Driscoll's (2007), I was actually doing quite a good job of reflecting! Completing this reflection has made me realise why I have found it so challenging to 'switch off' from work since the COVID-19 pandemic began, and that is primarily due to working from home the majority of the time for the first time in my career. I think this became a particular challenge for me due to a heavily increased workload and not finding a replacement for that 'walk home reflection' that I used to have and having no clear boundary between work and home life. There are several solutions to this, such as going for a walk after finishing work, switching where you physically work at home so that you can 'close the door' on your work or working at a completely different location all together but the key point is that I needed to reflect on why I was struggling with work–life boundaries, recognise that it was because I had always used my commute to reflect on and process my working day and find an appropriate solution to this.

Reflecting after the fact, as above, is known as 'reflecting *on* action' but as practitioners, what we sometimes struggle to identify is how much we 'reflect *in* action'. Reflecting on/in action relates to Schon's (1991) theory presented in his seminal book 'The Reflective Practitioner' (Schon, 1991). Reflection in action is something that we may do unconsciously and involves considering the situation at present, making a decision and acting in the moment. Some of the questions we may ask ourselves when reflecting in action could include:

- Have I been in this situation before?
- If so, what did I/we do to manage the situation?
- Did that go well?
- If so, will the same approach work in this situation?
- If not, what could we do differently?

We can reflect in action as a team by asking these questions aloud or asking 'what are our options?'. By doing this and then evaluating each option with our previous knowledge and experience is quintessentially, reflecting in action. As an experienced clinical practitioner, you may find it easy to quickly reflect in action and identify the best solution to a problem or situation. Still, you can support peers and those less experienced at reflecting in action by simply asking the above questions to them and supporting them to find the most appropriate answers.

Reflecting on our clinical practice is vitally important for all of the reasons discussed above. However, what is sometimes less considered is how we can develop our professional identities through reflection. This can be quite simply by asking the question 'what kind of practitioner do I want to be?'.

Activity

- Take some time to really consider that question; 'What kind of practitioner do you want to be?'
- How do you want your colleagues and clients to see you?
- How would you want junior staff or students to view you?

The response to the above activity will, of course, be very personal and individual, but many practitioners may want colleagues or clients to view them as kind, supportive, patient, knowledgeable and so on – all of which are positive attributes we would like to see in ourselves and in our colleagues. The next step is to think about your interactions. Do you think you have demonstrated those qualities within your interactions within the last week? If not, what do you think you could do differently next week? This may seem very simple, but this is very much how we develop our professional identities. Role-modelling is an important component of this, you may have a colleague you have worked with who you thought always demonstrated a caring approach, think of what they did and how they acted for you to see them that way and then think how you could replicate that as well. Role-modelling is something that we should always consider within our clinical practice – both in terms of looking to others for inspiration and as being a role model. I have been lucky enough to work with some incredible nurses during my career, and I have always tried to understand their approaches to be able to adopt them into my practice. If we consider all aspects of reflection, reflection in action, reflection on action, reflection on our professional identity and reflection in relation to role-modelling, we can see how reflection becomes a 360° all-encompassing aspect of our practice and professional identity.

References

Driscoll, J. (2007) *Practising clinical supervision: A reflective approach for healthcare professionals.* Edinburgh: Baillière Tindall Elsevier.

Gibbs, G. and Andrew, C. (2001) *Learning by doing: A guide to teaching and learning methods.* Geography Discipline Network.

The Nursing and Midwifery Council (n.d.) *Revalidation.* Available at: https://www.nmc.org.uk/revalidation/ (Accessed: 6 April 2023).

Schon, D.A. (1991) *The reflective practitioner: How professionals think in action.* Aldershot, U.K.: Ashgate.

CHAPTER 3

Resilience

You can't pour from an empty cup …

Resilience is a term that is referred to frequently in nursing, always emphasizing how important it is. When we consider the demands of working in healthcare, long shifts, high clinical caseloads and emotionally difficult work, we can understand why resilience is such an important consideration but what does it actually mean? How do we understand our resilience? How do we build resilience when we feel overwhelmed? This chapter will explore some of the key considerations around resilience, how we can understand our needs and build resilience for ourselves and others.

To over-simplify the term, resilience can be understood as our natural or learned defences to stressful situations and our ability to recover from these. We all have the capacity to deal with stress and stressors, but as we know, not all stressors are created equal! Holmes and Rahe in 1967 published their 'Social Readjustment Rating Scale' which assigned a numerical value to various stressful life events and in their research found that those with a score of over 300 were 80% more likely to experience health issues in the following two years (Holmes and Rahe, 1967). To contextualise this, the highest-ranking stressor was the death of a spouse, which scored 100 on the scale, retirement scored 45, and a 'minor violation of law' scored just 11. Many of us could look at the rating scale and question whether we would find that situation stressful, such as divorce (which scores 73). If someone were in an abusive marriage, for example, surely the more stressful thing would be to remain in the marriage? Retirement may be a significant life event but many of us eagerly await the day we can enjoy our retirement! There are many examples like this where individual perception would be a significant factor in the impact of different situations and scenarios however, the important factor with the Holmes and Rahe Scale (1967) is that it very much establishes a link between stress and health. Stress is a core concept in mental health nursing that will be returned to many times throughout this text, but the link between stress and health will be explored in much greater depth in the chapter focussing on 'the stress vulnerability model'.

Thriving in Mental Health Nursing, First Edition. Laura Duncan.
© 2025 John Wiley & Sons Ltd. Published 2025 by John Wiley & Sons Ltd.

When we consider 'what is resilience?' it is difficult to separate any definition from the concept of stress. Many consider resilience to be about coping with adverse experiences, whereas some view resilience as an inherent personality trait (Henshall, Davey and Jackson, 2020). However, this presents many challenges as an attitude to resilience as it implies that some are resilient and others are not and that this is an unchangeable status of being. Which, quite simply, it is not. Thinking of resilience as something that can have peaks and troughs leads to a more empathic understanding of ourselves and others. For example, think of a time when you have had a particularly bad night's sleep. How did that affect your mood? Did you find yourself more or less able to cope with stress the next day? Most people can empathise with how a single night's poor sleep can have a detrimental impact on your mood and stress levels, which then impacts your resilience. If we have been feeling stressed or overly tired, our resilience will be less than if we are generally feeling calm, supported and well rested. We can also reflect on when we were experiencing something challenging in our personal life, such as a bereavement or separation. That will have a significant impact on our work–life balance, we may not be able to work at all (particularly in the acute stages of a significant life event) and if we do continue to work/return to work, our quality and standard of work may not be of the same level as when we were not going through a difficult time in our personal life. After all, we are human and can only cope with so much stress, no one has unending resilience. Although we can develop strategies to identify when our resilience may be challenged and how to improve this, we must also recognise the importance of limits and boundaries. We frequently extend empathy to others but not ourselves.

Nursing as a whole is considered a stressful occupation; however; research (Foster et al., 2020) identifies that mental health nursing as a profession is particularly challenging due to factors such as increased levels of verbal and physical aggression and 'moral distress'. Moral distress can come from engaging in practices you ethically disagree with; even if you agree practically, it is the most appropriate action, such as utilising seclusion. Healthcare professionals in all areas and fields could be the victims of violence, abuse, or moral distress/injury, whilst we are focussing on mental health nursing, we must be mindful that we are not the only profession that experiences these challenging work environments. Mental health nurses reported that the most challenging workplace stressors were violence and aggression, followed by challenges with colleagues and organisational factors such as workload demands (Foster et al., 2020). This highlights the negative impact working in environments with high levels of violence and aggression has on clinicians and that ultimately, those who engaged in the research are effectively saying that their workload issues (which would include long shifts, staffing issues, high caseloads, etc.) is not as stressful or challenging as the presence or threat of violence and aggression. The second most common source of stress was collegiate, and nurses are frequently faced with adversity as part of their role, but it is surprising how frequently bullying appears within the literature as a significant source of stress for nurses (Henshall, Davey and Jackson, 2020; Foster et al., 2020). You would anticipate working in healthcare to be a supportive and kind environment but this appears to frequently not be the case. It is difficult to understand why bullying is so common within the profession and if in fact it is more common than in other professions. It is particularly shocking when you consider the current staffing crisis facing all fields of nursing and that feeling bullied or ostracised would be a strong motivator for nurses to leave the clinical area or even the profession. Increasing our personal resilience is obviously a positive factor within this; however, this highlights the importance of supporting our colleagues and peers to develop their resilience through supervision, compassionate practice and leadership. This, however, does not replace the need for organisations to improve support and healthy working environments for their staff (Henshall, Davey and Jackson, 2020). Developing improved resilience should be seen as a fundamental cultural and organisational issue (Henshall, Davey and Jackson, 2020) that should be a high priority for every organisation and leader within clinical services. Embedding positive attitudes and approaches to developing and improving resilience across teams and organisations would positively impact individual staff and may improve staff retention.

Now we've considered what resilience is and why it's important, we will now consider what it is not! Many professionals wear their resilience as a badge of honour, and while we should support and praise people for overcoming challenges and adversity, this can lead to a negative impact on that same individual and those around them. Imagine there has been a difficult incident on the ward, and one team member was injured. That team member may be very resilient and may feel they are fine and can continue with the shift; other members of the team may praise them for this and positively reinforce this behaviour. What if later they start experiencing more pain? If they've been praised for staying on shift and 'powering through', they may feel unable to say they are now struggling and need to go home. What about the other team members who were distressed by the incident but think that because they weren't physically injured, they can't say anything or ask for support as it will look like they aren't resilient? Presenteeism and 'hustle culture' are certainly not unique to nursing but the consequences within healthcare of presenteeism can be significant and severe. The definition of presenteeism is attending work when not physically or psychologically well enough to perform normally and one of the core reasons for presenteeism is the fear or concern of your colleague's being overloaded in your absence (Santos et al., 2022), however the evidence demonstrates that presenteeism causes decreased productivity, increased errors and poorer patient outcomes. One example of this is continuing to go to work with a cold. By doing so, you are risking passing this on to colleagues and patients. Now, your team all become unwell when this could have been avoided by staying at home when unwell. Logically, we all know we would not want our team members to come to work if they were physically unwell, but many still continue to do so. Physical health presenteeism has an obvious 'knock-on' effect but what about when someone is psychologically not well? Put simply, continuing to go to work when psychologically impaired (this could be from personal life or work–life stressors) can lead to burnout. Burnout is a crisis facing nursing currently, and ultimately, burnout starts as stress. Ongoing and chronic workplace stress leads to poor job satisfaction, distress and care standards becoming affected; staff can also experience vicarious traumatisation (Foster et al., 2020), and all of these factors can culminate to cause burnout.

In summary, resilience is not continuing to work regardless of what has happened or how you feel. One of the critical aspects of resilience is recognising your own boundaries and when you need to take time to rest and recover. Experiencing a difficult scenario that challenges our resilience is much like having a cold; by taking time to rest and recover at that moment will ultimately mean we feel better and able to continue with our work sooner and in a healthier manner.

It can be challenging to recognise our resilience; ultimately, this is part of our reflective skills. Developing our abilities in reflection will enable us to better understand and build our resilience throughout our careers and this should be seen as an ongoing commitment such as continuous professional development and lifelong learning.

Activity

- Think about something that you found mildly challenging in your work life in recent months; take some time to make notes on what it was about that situation/scenario that you found challenging and how you overcame this.
- Imagine yourself 10 years ago, where were you? Were you at school? University? Working?
- How would the recent scenario have affected the you of 10 years ago?
- How do you think you would have felt? Would you have managed the situation in the same way? Would you have found it more challenging? Would you have had more of an emotional response?

When undertaking that activity, many people would feel that the 'them of 10 years ago' possibly wouldn't have handled the situation as well/competently/efficiently as present-day them. This is because age and experience do naturally build our resilience, and it is important for us to recognise how our resilience has developed. Research supports this as younger mental health nurses appear to be more adversely affected by stressors than those who are older and more experienced in the field (Foster et al., 2020) which could account for the high attrition rate for early career nurses and demonstrates the importance of providing better support for newly qualified nurses in particular. The fact that resilience builds with experience is a valuable takeaway, as many may feel that if they feel un-resilient, that that will never change.

To improve our resilience, we need to reflect on when we have felt un-resilient. What was happening? What was the situation or scenario, and was this an ongoing feeling over a period of time or something you felt for a brief period? We may find that upon reflection, we identify that similar scenarios challenge our resilience and these will be unique to each individual. Some may find working with a client who has recently harmed themselves very challenging and upsetting, for example, and if we can identify that self-harm is an area that we find challenging then we can focus specifically on this and develop strategies such as ensuring that there is a de-brief with a colleague you are comfortable with following any incidents that involve self-harm. Our mindset is also crucial to identifying and developing our resilience, and research suggests that some of the factors and attributes that can improve resilience are seeing challenges as an opportunity, accepting our limits, having a good sense of humour and crucially, accepting help from others (McDermott et al., 2020). All of these factors are things we can identify and improve on if we want to strengthen our resilience (yes, even humour!). They inherently need our skills in reflection to help us identify which ones we could improve and when. Being goal orientated in our work and studies can also aid with resilience (McDermott et al., 2020) as this can help focus our mindset on recognising that stress and challenges are temporary and, if we want to achieve our goals, must be overcome.

Accepting help from others and recognising when to ask for help is an important aspect of improving our resilience. Still, to develop positive cultures in working environments then there must be reciprocity in that we offer that support to our peers and colleagues as well. We need to recognise that mental health nursing is a stressful profession, and interestingly, in Foster et al.'s research (2020), they found that no mental health nurse reported zero workplace stressors; in fact, the majority reported 15 or more stressors, and experiencing verbal aggression was reported by 98% of respondents. Suicide and self-harming behaviour were very prominent stressors in Foster et al.'s (2020) findings and were particularly emotionally demanding and distressing for mental health nurses. This highlights the importance of effective and consistent strategies to support nurses within their roles however even when there are good support mechanisms in place for clinical staff such as reflective practice and supervision, these are frequently sacrificed when there is a clinical issue (Henshall, Davey and Jackson, 2020) such as staffing shortfalls or an incident. Whilst this may sometimes be necessary when there is an immediate issue, if they are not promptly rescheduled, it further evidences that the needs of staff are sometimes at the bottom of the priority list in clinical areas leaving people feeling devalued and unsupported. As individuals, our crucial role within this should be to recognise when these supportive mechanisms, such as supervision, are being missed, offer ad hoc support to our team members, and escalate our concerns to our seniors if this is a consistent and persistent issue within our clinical team. This does not just apply to line-management arrangements; we do not need to be senior to a colleague to offer ad hoc or informal supervision to support their emotional or well-being needs.

Consideration, support and training specifically around resilience should begin during nurse education, particularly when we consider that nursing students face many stressors whilst undertaking their studies including intensive academic and practical workloads in clinical practice (Drach-Zahavy et al., 2021) and experienced nurses can sometimes forget how challenging undertaking a nursing programme truly is. Many have argued the need for specific focus and training on resilience within nurse education (McDermott et al., 2020), and that during education, nurse academics have a specific role in providing resilience-related learning, being supportive to nursing students during stressful situations, and supporting students in reflecting on challenges positively and constructively. Suppose we were to embed resilience training throughout preregistration nursing programmes collectively, we may see significant benefits in terms of retention of student nurses in the first instance but then more resilient nurses who are better prepared for the profession's challenges. This may also lead to a more supportive workforce overall, which would improve the experience of not only the clinical team but also service users as well as the overall well-being of the nursing workforce is crucial to their capacity to provide safe, person-centred and effective care (Foster et al., 2020).

Vignette

To protect the identities of those involved, I will be deliberately vague about some of the details of the scenario from my clinical practice. This vignette is provided to support linking theory to practice and share a reflective account that will hopefully help you in your own reflections.

I had only been qualified as a nurse for about 18 months when I moved teams, and due to some fairly complex contractual reasons, I was working within a team who were all from a different organisation to me, meaning they had no management responsibilities over me. I have always been a good team player and thrived in inpatient teams but this team was very small and well established before I had started there. I have reflected upon my early days/weeks/months there many times and have frequently asked myself, 'What would I have done differently?' and each time, I have drawn a blank. The reason for that is not because I see myself as the perfect practitioner but instead because I approached that team with kindness and openness and that is simply something that I will not regret. I worked in that team for a year in total and it was the absolute worst year of my career. One member of that team would be fine to work with; nothing would have happened and nothing would have been said, but then a few hours later, I would get a call from my line manager telling me she had made a complaint against me for something that had no basis in fact. I have never and will never understand her motivations and it took me a very long time (and several counselling sessions!) to name it as bullying.

All of the accusations she made were bizarre and made little/no sense. They included examples such as me saying 'as it's quiet, I might pop down to introduce myself to "x" team as my manager told me to do that when I could, is that ok with you?', her replying 'yes that's fine, I did that too when I first started here' and then my manager later called me after she called her manager, who called my manager to ask why I'd said I was going to work in a different team, in a different location. Obviously, I hadn't said that as that wasn't the case, she knew that wasn't what was said but chose to make a complaint about it for what reason? Her lies and malicious complaints led to me frequently being shouted at first thing in the morning by her line manager, often before I'd even managed to take my coat off.

I explained the situation to my manager (who was also somewhat fed up with the constant phone calls!), who was supportive and told me she was escalating the matter further. Every month at my line-management supervision, I begged to be transferred, but there was always a reason that couldn't be facilitated.

This went on for a year and had an incredibly negative impact on my well-being and mental health. I never felt comfortable or that I could relax, I was watching every word I said and tried to guess how it could be misinterpreted or manipulated and was constantly on edge. That workplace was a 2-hour commute via train, and most nights, I would be sobbing on the train home. The situation culminated in her calling me on a day off and basically implying that I was going to get arrested as a client I had assessed had been arrested and named me as the reason they hadn't complied with their bail conditions. Despite experiencing her lies for a year, it didn't occur to me that this was also a lie, so before calling the police officer who wanted to speak to me 'and go to the station for an interview' I called my line manager for advice. She calmed me down and advised me to call the police officer and ask how I could help, and we would go from there. I did that, and they asked me some questions about this client if I had any acute concerns, etc., and after about 15 minutes, I asked if I was in trouble or needed to come to the station. The officer was shocked because what had actually happened was that they told my colleague that they were aware I'd put a robust support package in place and they would just like to ask me about it and if there were any other services the client should be referred to.

The situation continued deteriorating until I was eventually moved to a different environment to work alongside a new team that was very supportive and professional.

So, what does this mean about my resilience? Well, first, I'd suggest I was very resilient to continue to show up and do my job when working in an environment as toxic and hostile as that!

Second, I learned some very valuable lessons that I have taken forward in the rest of my career. When I reflect back on how young I was, how newly qualified and inexperienced (from the perspective of myself now) I was, I am amazed at how professionally I handled that situation. I never retaliated; I continued to behave like a professional; I was respectful and utilised the appropriate mechanisms, such as my management team and supervision arrangements. I cried, a lot, but always outside of the environment. Never letting her see how upset and distressed I was will always be a source of pride.

Reflecting on how I actually was incredibly resilient to continue functioning in the face of such challenges has made me appraise my ability to cope with future issues more positively. I have frequently found myself thinking 'well it's not as bad as "x" that's for sure!' and knowing that I would ultimately be fine. It did take me time and an excellent counsellor to be able to frame it as an experience that I learned and grew from and could ultimately be proud of myself for.

There could have been an alternative scenario (and it absolutely did cross my mind at times) where I left the profession. I think if I hadn't have had such positive experiences as a support worker before I undertook my nurse training, the balance could have very much shifted for me to feel that nursing was not the profession for me. Luckily, I had enough background and experience to recognise that that was not normal for Mental Health services, and I was able to move to another team who were lovely human beings that recognised what I had been through and could not have been more supportive.

If I were to experience the same situation now, over a decade later, I'd like to think I would feel more secure in asserting myself and advocating for myself. I generally feel much more confident in challenging others than I did, and I think that can be a very difficult concept for those of us who don't like confrontation! I certainly don't think it would happen in the same manner and absolutely not for a year! The other important takeaway for me is that it has made me quite sensitive to how others may feel when new to a team or environment and that I would never, ever want anyone to think that I had treated them poorly or caused them distress. Due to this, I try to approach even difficult conversations in a positive and friendly way and frequently use humour. Ultimately, even though it was an incredibly difficult experience to live through, I can reflect on my resiliency now, and seeing that as a positive further improves my resilience. It has also made me a more thoughtful and considerate practitioner throughout my career.

In summary, we all have natural levels of resilience and will respond to stress differently. If our resilience is challenged, we need to seek support and help actively. We can reflect on our levels of resilience to help build this further, and we should be supporting our colleagues to seek help when needed and feel comfortable to acknowledge when their resilience is tested.

References

Drach-Zahavy, A. et al. (2021) 'A multi-level examination of nursing students' resilience in the face of the Covid-19 outbreak: A cross-sectional design', *Journal of Advanced Nursing*, 78(1), pp. 109–120. doi:10.1111/jan.14951.

Foster, K., Roche, M., Giandinoto, J., Platania-Phung, C. and Furness, T. (2020). Mental health matters: A cross-sectional study of mental health nurses' health-related quality of life and work-related stressors. *International Journal of Mental Health Nursing*, 30(3). https://doi.org/10.1111/inm.12823.

Henshall, C., Davey, Z. and Jackson, D. (2020) 'Nursing resilience interventions-a way forward in challenging healthcare territories', *Journal of Clinical Nursing*, doi:10.1111/jocn.15276.

Holmes, T.H. and Rahe, R.H. (1967). The social readjustment rating scale. *Journal of Psychosomatic Research*, [online] 11(2), pp. 213–218. https://doi.org/10.1016/0022-3999(67)90010-4.

Mcdermott, R.C. et al. (2020) 'Nursing students' resilience, depression, well-being, and academic distress: Testing a moderated mediation model', *Journal of Advanced Nursing*, 76(12), pp. 3385–3397. doi:10.1111/jan.14531.

Santos, B. da S., Rocha, F.L.R., Bortolini, J., Terra, F. de S. and Valim, M.D. (2022). Factors associated with presenteeism in nursing workers. *Revista Brasileira de Enfermagem*, 75(1). https://doi.org/10.1590/0034-7167-2020-1290.

CHAPTER 4

Emotional Intelligence

Emotional intelligence is the ability to perceive, understand, process, regulate and express emotion in a way that facilitates thought and growth (Sánchez-Núñez et al., 2020). Emotional intelligence relates to being able to recognise and monitor your own feelings, evaluate them and then use the information to make decisions about your thinking and actions (Van Dusseldorp, Van Meijel and Derksen, 2011). It is about our ability to respond rather than react to our feelings and use them productively moving forward. Emotional intelligence is not about not having or experiencing emotional responses, it is actually the opposite! It is about being able to acknowledge you have had an emotional response, understand why and what has caused it and utilise that information to make an informed decision about what to do next. High levels of emotional intelligence are linked to improved well-being, life satisfaction and better leadership skills (Shami, Tareh and Taran, 2017). Emotional intelligence is strongly impacted through parental behaviour and role modelling during childhood and adolescence (Sánchez-Núñez et al., 2020). This means that our emotional intelligence tends to be similar to that of our parents and family members but can be influenced by anyone in our social circles. High levels of emotional intelligence are linked to increased resilience, providing protection from stress and improved adaptability (Sánchez-Núñez et al., 2020). Emotional intelligence is strongly linked to self-awareness, self-control and empathy (Van Dusseldorp, Van Meijel and Derksen, 2011). It is implicitly linked to the concept of reflection. It forms a core part of how we reflect, particularly when we reflect on the emotional impact of a situation or scenario. Emotional intelligence is not about 'head vs. heart' but instead about combining emotion with intelligence in decision-making and problem-solving (Akerjordet and Severinsson, 2004). Those who lack emotional clarity have higher rates of anxiety and stress, and research suggests that those with mental health issues tend to have lower levels of emotional intelligence (Sánchez-Núñez et al., 2020). This means that those engaging with mental health services may have difficulties with emotional intelligence and understanding how their emotions impact them and their decision-making, highlighting the importance of role-modelling good emotional intelligence to those in our care.

Self-awareness is at the core of emotional intelligence and crucial to mental health nursing (Akerjordet and Severinsson, 2004). Emotional intelligence in healthcare professionals helps

Thriving in Mental Health Nursing, First Edition. Laura Duncan.
© 2025 John Wiley & Sons Ltd. Published 2025 by John Wiley & Sons Ltd.

them manage their own emotions when working with clients who have experienced trauma (MacLaren, 2024). Working in health and social care in any context is an emotionally challenging role, but this is particularly true for mental health professionals who will be exposed daily to discussions of trauma and traumatic incidents, highlighting the importance of understanding emotional intelligence to be able to manage our emotional responses in a productive and healthy way. It is imperative for mental health professionals to be able to differentiate between their own emotions and the emotions of their clients (Akerjordet and Severinsson, 2004). However, it can be very challenging to do this, and we will often feel emotions without understanding why or where they came from. Clients who have emotional regulation difficulties, in particular, can lead clinicians 'holding' those feelings, but being able to understand that 'this is not my emotion' can be helpful in terms of processing and moving forward. Mental health professionals' emotional response and ability to manage their own emotions can directly impact therapeutic relationships (Van Dusseldorp, Van Meijel and Derksen, 2011). If a clinician were struggling to manage their emotions and became angry or tearful during an interaction, it is clear how this could impact a therapeutic relationship negatively.

Mental health nurses tend to have above-average levels of emotional intelligence (Van Dusseldorp, Van Meijel and Derksen, 2011). This is likely due to mental health nurses focussing on thoughts and feelings as part of their everyday roles, therefore, having a greater understanding of how feelings can impact behaviour more clearly than those outside of mental health as a profession. Emotional intelligence can be developed and improved (Van Dusseldorp, Van Meijel and Derksen, 2011). This is an important consideration as we should be striving as clinicians to build our knowledge and skills in all arenas. The impact of emotional intelligence is not only on our clinical skills but also on our well-being; it highlights the need to actively try to improve levels of emotional intelligence not only for ourselves but also for our colleagues. Clinical supervision and reflection can help us develop greater emotional intelligence (Akerjordet and Severinsson, 2004). Reflection is particularly important, and having the space within clinical supervision to express our emotions and how they have impacted us and our decision-making is crucial to enhancing our emotional intelligence as clinicians. Embedding emotional intelligence training and understanding in healthcare education could have positive outcomes in terms of strengthening therapeutic relationships, the quality of care provided and reducing stress for clinicians (Van Dusseldorp, Van Meijel and Derksen, 2011). Emotional intelligence should be considered early in the careers of clinicians as it is not only important for developing clinical skills and enhancing therapeutic relationships but it would also be a protective factor for healthcare professionals in reducing stress, poor job satisfaction and burnout.

Activity

Although we may already have excellent emotional intelligence, there is always room for improvement! Below are some tips for how we can improve our emotional intelligence:

- Pay attention to your feelings; try to name them and see if you can feel them within your body. For example, it may be 'worry' and you can feel it in your chest or 'sadness' in your stomach.

- Try to understand why you have that feeling; is it because of something someone said to you or their behaviour? Has it come from somewhere else that isn't directly happening right now?
- Think about your reaction to the feeling. Has it made you want to do something in a particular way? Why do you think that is? What has prompted that desire to react?
- Consider whether your impulse to react will have the desired outcome. Reacting to a feeling of panic in an emergency could be the absolute right thing to do but reacting when feeling angry is unlikely to have a positive outcome.
- Consider your opinions. If you have a strong opinion about a scenario or situation, why is that? Is that linked to an emotional response?
- Reflect on how your feelings have impacted your actions; this is part of everything we do, so you should not feel critical or negative.
- Check your intuition. Healthcare professionals frequently have an intuition that something is wrong or needs to happen; this is usually closely linked to an emotion we have felt; therefore, see if you can see any patterns.
- Recognise the emotions of others. Just as we will have emotional responses, so will those around us. Trying to think of how their emotions are impacting their behaviour can be helpful in understanding how to support them or move forward.
- Listen to feedback. Sometimes, we may not recognise an emotion driving our behaviour or response to situations, so if someone offers you feedback, try to take it open-mindedly.

Case Study

Kyle is a 21-year-old female who has just been admitted to an inpatient mental health unit. Kyle has been supported by Child and Adolescent Mental Health Services (CAMHS) since she was 14 years old after her father found that she was engaging in self-injurious behaviour by cutting herself. Kyle's mother passed away when she was 8 years old. Kyle found the transition to adult services very difficult as she had developed a strong therapeutic relationship with her CAMHS care coordinator. It was included in her care notes that Kyle was sexually abused as a child by a babysitter, and this seems to have precipitated her cutting behaviour. She was later diagnosed with anxiety, and at 18 was diagnosed with emotionally unstable personality disorder. Kyle has not had contact with her father or any other member of her family in several years as she blames her father for employing the babysitter who sexually abused her. Kyle now lives in supported accommodation and was admitted to the inpatient unit after being found with a ligature tied around her neck.

Take some time now to reflect on the information above and answer the following questions:

- Have you had an emotional response to Kyle's background?
- If so, what emotion are you feeling?
- What do your feelings make you think about the next steps for Kyle or how you would approach the situation?

Kyle has been on the ward for two hours and is very upset. She has been hostile to anyone who tries to speak to her, and when you tried to approach her, she swore at you and told you to go away. Your colleague tried to approach her a few minutes later, and she spat at him, shouting and swearing for him to leave her alone and let her just kill herself. Your colleague has returned to the office and called Kyle 'that little bitch'.

- What are your feelings and emotions at this moment?
- What do you think your colleague is feeling?

- How would you respond to your colleague after thinking about his feelings?
- What actions would you want to take next?

You tell your colleague that you understand that it's horrible to be spat at and that he is understandably having an emotional reaction to that, but he needs to be mindful of his language and can't call a client names. He takes a breath and tells you that you are right, he shouldn't have said that and didn't mean it. He says that he really can't stand being spat at and it made him feel so angry in the moment. You suggest to your colleague that he take a break and go off the ward for a few minutes to gather his thoughts and process his feelings. He agrees and says he'll be back in 10 minutes when he's calmed down.

You decide to try to approach Kyle again, knock on the door to her room and she swears at you again. You open the door and say that you would just ask if she wanted a drink. Kyle stares at you and then says 'Tea, two sugars' bluntly. You smile and say 'ok' before walking away to make her the drink. You make one for yourself, and when you return, offer Kyle the tea; she says thank you very curtly and you ask if it would be ok to join her for a few minutes. She shrugs and doesn't answer.

- What are your feelings at this moment?
- What do you think Kyle is feeling up until this point?
- How is this information going to inform your next actions?

You sit silently for a few minutes, drinking your tea, Kyle does the same. You perceive that she seems a little calmer. You have noticed that she has a Disney character on her phone case, and you think this could be an excellent way to break the ice. You ask her if it is Stitch (from the film 'Lilo and Stitch') on her phone case, and she looks at you and nods. You say 'I love Stitch, he's one of my faves too'. Kyle says she thinks he's the best and has always loved the film. You continue to talk about Disney films while you drink your tea, and Kyle seems to be lot calmer than she was previously.

- How are you feeling at this point?
- What do you think Kyle might be feeling?
- How do you think this engagement has impacted your therapeutic relationship with Kyle?

You tell Kyle that you know she hasn't been here before, so it must be difficult not knowing where you are or who anyone is. Kyle looks tearful and nods. You reassure her that you and the rest of the team are here to help her, and she nods again. You tell Kyle that it's ok and normal to be upset or distressed, but it's not ok to spit at people, and so moving forward, if she wants time alone, then that's ok, but she can't spit at people. Kyle looks at you and doesn't speak for a moment. She is still tearful, but you can't tell whether she is upset or angry. After a few seconds, Kyle says 'fine. I get it but I don't want any men in my room. If they come in my room then I'm going to defend myself'. You explain gently that you can share her request with the team but that there are male staff who are here to support her. You advise that when she's settled, you can think together about the best way forward with the whole team, and Kyle nods. Kyle tells you she's tired and wants to have a nap; you tell her that sounds like a good plan and if she needs anything, she can come and find you. Kyle nods and lies down.

Reflect one last time on the final aspect of the scenario.

- What do you think your emotional response would be to Kyle's statements?
- How do you think Kyle felt during your time in her room?
- Do you think raising the spitting incident at that time was appropriate? What other considerations would you have made?
- How do you think you would have felt leaving the room?

As we can see from this scenario, in a concise time, there were a lot of emotions! You were considering and responding to the emotions of yourself, Kyle and your colleague. In the scenario, we can see that your colleague had a strong emotional reaction that impacted their behaviour in a way that wasn't appropriate. By acknowledging his feelings and helping him to reflect in the moment, he could see his emotions had impacted his behaviour negatively and he took a break to be able to manage them more appropriately. This is not to say that he has poor emotional intelligence because we will all have moments when our emotions are overwhelming or may impact our response negatively; he demonstrated good emotional intelligence in being able to reflect on the moment and acknowledge how his feelings had affected him and that he needed some time to address this. You also helped Kyle to reflect on her emotions and actions but this was more complex due to not having previously had a relationship with Kyle like you did with your colleague. In the scenario, you took time to try to calm the situation down and start to develop a therapeutic relationship by finding something of interest for Kyle to discuss. You waited until some rapport had been established and Kyle's emotions appeared less intense before addressing her behaviour with her. She was able to make some steps forward in that interaction, and you were able to establish information that could be important not only for your therapeutic relationship with Kyle but also for how the team works with and supports her. You not only supported Kyle and your colleague but also helped them to develop their emotional intelligence, and by reflecting on your own emotional responses, you are able to improve yourself as well.

As we can see, emotional intelligence impacts everything we do as mental health professionals. Having good emotional intelligence helps us not only to work therapeutically with clients but also to safeguard ourselves from stress and burnout. Acknowledging our emotions and how they affect and influence us is an important skill that we should be continuously striving to improve.

References

Akerjordet, K. and Severinsson, E. (2004) 'Emotional intelligence in mental health nurses talking about practice'. *International Journal of Mental Health Nursing*, 13(3), pp. 164–170. doi:10.1111/j.1440-0979.2004.0328.x.

Maclaren, J. (2024) 'Barriers to trauma-informed care include unsafe environments and mental health nurses' lack of emotional intelligence'. *Evidence Based Nursing/Evidence-Based Nursing*, p.ebnurs-103998. doi:10.1136/ebnurs-2024-103998.

Sánchez-Núñez, M.T., García-Rubio, N., Fernández-Berrocal, P. and Latorre, J.M. (2020) 'Emotional intelligence and mental health in the family: The influence of emotional intelligence perceived by parents and children'. *International Journal of Environmental Research and Public Health*, 17(17), p. 6255. doi:10.3390/ijerph17176255.

Shami, R., Tareh, M. and Taran, H. (2017) 'Identifying the relationship among teacher's mental health and emotional intelligence and their burnout'. *Independent Journal of Management & Production*, 8(1), pp. 124–143. doi:10.14807/ijmp.v8i1.513.

van Dusseldorp, L.R., van Meijel, B.K. and Derksen, J.J. (2011) 'Emotional intelligence of mental health nurses'. *Journal of Clinical Nursing*, 20(3–4), pp. 555–562. doi:10.1111/j.1365-2702.2009.03120.x.

CHAPTER 5

Listening and Communication Skills

Effective communication is crucial within clinical care settings (Pidano, Padukkavidana and Honigfeld, 2017). Communication is understood as the exchange of both verbal and nonverbal information (Bramhall, 2014). Communication includes not only what we say and how we say it in terms of our tone, volume, and pitch but also our body language, eye contact and facial expressions. Written communication is vital in all healthcare settings as it is the primary way of sharing important information with staff and service users, and so ensuring that our written documentation is clear, accurate and appropriate is of vital importance. When we consider how much of a clinician's role is focussed on the transmission of information, communication skills are arguably one of the most important factors for nurses (Baghbanzadeh and Sobhi, 2021).

Communication is vital to have positive caring relationships and good teamwork (Bramhall, 2014). We frequently focus on communication skills in terms of our therapeutic relationships with clients, but we sometimes forget that effective teamwork and positive inter-colleague relationships are also based on good communication skills. When considering clients, person-centred communication is associated with increased rates of satisfaction (Pidano, Padukkavidana and Honigfeld, 2017). This means that as clinicians, we need to adapt our communication style to suit the client. There can be significant adverse outcomes from poor or ineffective communication, including worsening of symptoms or more restrictive measures being used, such as hospitalisation (Papageorgiou, Loke and Fromage, 2017) when we don't precisely understand a client's feelings, needs or preferences. Clients with conditions such as schizophrenia can find it difficult to communicate with clinicians effectively and vice versa (Papageorgiou, Loke and Fromage, 2017). There can be many factors that impact someone's communication style or needs, including experiencing a mental health condition, such as schizophrenia or being in distress – more generally speaking – but also if a client has specific social and communication difficulties. Someone with learning difficulties may need information to be communicated in a simplified manner or prefer to use other communication formats, such as pictures or sign language. If someone has

Thriving in Mental Health Nursing, First Edition. Laura Duncan.
© 2025 John Wiley & Sons Ltd. Published 2025 by John Wiley & Sons Ltd.

autistic spectrum disorder, they may experience sensory difficulties that make it difficult for them to communicate if there is lots of noise, or they may need more literal language to be used rather than euphemisms. Someone may experience hearing or vision loss that can significantly impact how communication is perceived, or there may be language or cultural barriers. The variety and spectrum of communication needs are potentially unending, which highlights the importance of the clinician needing to understand the client and their specific communication style and preferences for effective communication. Ultimately, the onus is on clinicians to ensure that information can be understood by the client effectively (Bramhall, 2014).

Listening is a core skill within mental health practice (Aadam, Poon and Fernandez, 2023); however, we don't frequently reflect on our listening skills. Listening should be focussed on making sense of the other person's experience and not on formulating a response (Aadam, Poon and Fernandez, 2023). It can be challenging when engaging with someone not to try to consider what to say or do next with the information provided, which is why we need to focus on active listening skills during our therapeutic interactions. Even when experiencing periods of distress, clients who felt that nurses had actively listened and demonstrated compassion feel more positive about their experiences of receiving care (Bramhall, 2014). This highlights that simply feeling 'heard' can be therapeutic within itself and a positive experience. Service Users report feeling disempowered and diminished when they are not listened to by clinicians (Aadam, Poon and Fernandez, 2023), and this can add to feelings of frustration, which can significantly damage the therapeutic relationship. Effective listening not only helps our understanding of a client's needs but it helps us to analyse information appropriately and create care plans (Aadam, Poon and Fernandez, 2023). Listening effectively to truly understand the person's experience and feelings helps us formulate our clinical opinion and create a pathway towards recovery. Ensuring that clients feel comfortable in expressing their thoughts and feelings leads to improved communication sharing and increased disclosure of information. Three factors are strongly associated with greater levels of disclosure, and those are asking questions relating to psychosocial issues, listening attentively and making supportive statements (Pidano, Padukkavidana and Honigfeld, 2017). Focussing on the whole person by asking questions around their psychosocial needs rather than just clinical symptoms is important in building relationships and conducting a holistic assessment that builds a clear picture of the person and their life. Active listening skills involve demonstrating that you have heard and understood by reframing, clarifying and asking questions to ensure you have effectively understood (Aadam, Poon and Fernandez, 2023). Active listening skills, including mirroring back and paraphrasing, can feel uncomfortable when we are first learning and utilising these skills. However, finding comfortable ways to do so means that our listening skills become heightened and more confident over time. Feeling listened to is strongly linked to recovery and feeling safe for Service Users (Aadam, Poon and Fernandez, 2023). Our goal as clinicians should always be towards recovery and clients feeling comfortable within our care and so this highlights the importance of effective listening skills to ensure we meet those goals.

Therapeutic communication skills are core to mental health nursing practice and should be a key focus throughout education and training (Fitzgerald, 2020) and a clinician's career.

Clinical staff can learn significant communication skills from role-modelling (Bramhall, 2014). Role-modelling is an important consideration for all clinical skills and identifying colleagues who demonstrate effective listening and communication skills and trying to understand how they utilise these skills practically can advance our clinical skills significantly. Listening is a skill that can be developed and improved upon through reflection (Aadam, Poon and Fernandez, 2023). Reflection is ultimately how we understand where our skill level currently is and where we would like to develop, and so it is imperative not only for our listening and communication skills but in every aspect of our roles. Role-play is a common method used to enhance learning when undertaking training or education. The benefit of role-play is that learners can take the place of the service user and experience what it may feel like to be in that position, the learner can also practice their clinical skills in a supportive environment where it is ok to make mistakes or not be perfect. This can help clinicians to develop empathy as well as the clinical skills that the role-play is focussed on, and receiving feedback when in the role of the clinician can help us to understand how others perceive our skills. Evidence shows that using role-play during education can help to improve therapeutic and communication skills for Mental Health students (Rønning and Bjørkly, 2019). While education and training can be very skills focussed, research has shown that training that focuses on interaction style, attitude and skills has the most significant positive impact on communication skills and clinical outcomes (Wissow et al., 2011). Reflecting on how we came across to others and their perception of our clinical skills and our attitude towards them can be a powerful tool in developing our therapeutic communication and listening skills. In summary, good communication skills improve care outcomes for clients (Bramhall, 2014), which is why we must focus on them throughout our career. Good communication and listening skills not only benefit clients though as nurses with good communication skills report improved quality of life and a lower incidence of depression (Baghbanzadeh and Sobhi, 2021). There could be many factors that contribute to these findings, but if we consider a nurse with excellent communication and listening skills, they are more likely to have positive therapeutic and inter-professional relationships and can express their thoughts and needs clearly and understandably, which would help improve their job satisfaction in particular. Good communication and listening skills not only help us to understand but to be understood.

Activity

Take some time to think about a time in your life where you felt 'unheard'. It can be an example from your personal or professional life.

- What was the situation?
- What were you trying to communicate?
- What did the person you were communicating with do that made you feel unheard?
  - Was it their body language?
  - Did they interrupt you?
  - Did they misinterpret the point of what you were saying?

- How did that make you feel?
- How would you tell the person how you felt during that interaction?

When we reflect on a situation where we may have felt unheard, it can help us determine specific actions or behaviours that may have led to this. When we can understand from our perspective what may make us feel unheard, we can then utilise this information to change our actions and behaviours.

Case Study

Jessie is a 20-year-old female. She has been admitted to an inpatient mental health unit for the first time after having suicidal thoughts. She has never had contact with mental health services before, and there is very little information about Jessie from the handover. The assessment that took place before her admission mainly gives her demographic information and says that she was expressing severe suicidal thoughts and intent and was very withdrawn. You are Jessie's named nurse and are about to undertake your first conversation with her.

- What information do you think you need to gather within this conversation?
- What are your main considerations for your communication style at this moment?

You invite Jessie into a quiet room on the ward, and she agrees, comes in, and takes a seat. You sit in a chair opposite her. Jessie is looking at the floor; her shoulders are hunched forward and her hands are tightly clenched in her lap.

- What are your immediate thoughts on Jessie's body language?

You introduce yourself to Jessie and explain that you will be her named nurse throughout her admission. She nods but does not look up. You explain that you are here to support Jessie and would like to get to know her better and understand what has been happening to her. She nods again.

- What would you do next?

The conversation goes as follows, (...) indicates a pause.

You: I understand this is your first time on a ward like this, is that correct?
Jessie: mmm-hmm
You: How are you finding it?
Jessie: Erm ... ok ... I suppose
You: ok?
Jessie: Ye, it's difficult. It's really loud.
You: It definitely can be quite loud sometimes
Jessie: Ye, there's lots of shouting
You: How does the shouting make you feel?
Jessie: erm ... Scared to be honest. I'm not used to it and it's just, I dunno ... a bit frightening
You: I can understand that. Is there anything I can do that might make you feel more comfortable?
Jessie: I don't know. I think I just want to go home.
You: I understand, it can be really difficult being in a new environment, particularly when it feels frightening. Tell me about home, do you live with anyone?

Jessie: I did live with my boyfriend
You: ... Did? Do you not live with him anymore?
Jessie: No. He moved out last week.
You: Is that something that you wanted to happen?
Jessie: No, I didn't want to break up, he did and just left me out of nowhere.
You: I'm so sorry Jessie, that must be really difficult
Jessie: Ye, I feel so stupid because I know it's just a boyfriend but I don't have anyone else and so, what's the point you know?
You: Why would you say that you feel stupid?
Jessie: Because there are bigger problems in the world, you know what I mean?
You: well, maybe but that doesn't make your problems any smaller does it?
Jessie: I suppose not. ...
You: So how have you been feeling recently?
Jessie: Pretty shit to be honest
You: Has that been the case since the breakup or were you feeling bad before that?
Jessie: Before. It's basically why he left me.
You: You think he left because you were feeling low?
Jessie: Ye, he said he couldn't stand living with 'a miserable bitch' anymore
You: That must have been a pretty hurtful thing to hear
Jessie: Ye that was actually quite mild for him to be honest
You: What do you mean?
Jessie: He used to call me all sorts, all the time. I couldn't do anything right. Literally anything I tried to do was wrong.
You: That sounds really bad. Did you ever talk to anyone else about this?
Jessie: No. I basically fell out with all my friends and family so it was just him, I didn't have anyone else to talk to
You: That sounds really lonely.
Jessie: Ye, it is. But it's my own fault.
You: What makes you say that?
Jessie: Well he didn't like me going out with my friends, so I just cut them all off and told them I didn't want to see them anymore
You: Did you want to keep seeing them?
Jessie: Ye of course. Most of them had been my mates since we were tiny, they were like sisters to me
You: That's really tough. Have you spoken to any of them recently?
Jessie: No. I thought about reaching out after he broke up with me, but I figured they wouldn't want to speak to me
You: Why do you think that?
Jessie: I dunno. I just cut them off and blocked them, why would they want to speak to me?
You: OK well what if you did reach out, what do you think the worst thing that could happen would be?
Jessie: That they'd ignore me or tell me how shit a friend I am?
You: OK and do you think that would be better or worse than the situation now?
Jessie: I dunno. What if they hate me?
You: What if they don't?
Jessie: Ye maybe if I explained and said I was sorry, they might talk to me again?
You: I think that sounds like a good step to take, what do you think?

Jessie: Ye, I think I will. We were always so close and they've messed up before too and we've always gotten over it so ye... maybe they will forgive me?

You: I think from what you've said, they're really important people in your life and you've been feeling really low and isolated recently so trying to get back in touch could be a really good step but it's your decision, you have to do what you think is best

Jessie: Ye, I'm going to message them, would you help me write the message? I want to make sure it's good and that I explain properly

You: Of course

Jessie: I'll go grab my phone

Throughout the aforementioned 5-minute discussion, Jessie began making eye contact. At the last minute, she sat up straighter, and her posture seemed more open. She was smiling as she left to get her phone.

In the conversation above, this is the first conversation between you and Jessie so the key focus should be to make Jessie feel comfortable and build rapport. There are clear verbal signals within the conversation that Jessie's mood has been bad for some time and that her boyfriend was not kind to her and could possibly have been abusive. Helping Jessie think about her friends and reaching out to them has had a clear and immediate positive impact on her mood and supporting her to make contact with them has helped to develop your therapeutic relationship as Jessie is developing trust in you to help and support her. Our initial contact does not need to be focussed on the heavy topics of why they may have been admitted or referred into services but should be focussed on positive relationship building.

Look at the conversation above and consider the following:

- Did your character use open-ended questions throughout?
- Where did your character demonstrate empathy?
- Did your character encourage Jessie to reflect at any point?
- Did your character push Jessie into talking about her thoughts and feelings?
- How do you think Jessie would have perceived your character?
- Do you think this was a positive interaction?
- What would you have done differently?
- What tone did you read the conversation in? Does your perception change if you alter the tone?
- What did you picture your body language being? Does the interaction change if your body language is different?

As you can see, not all questions used were 'open questions' as sometimes that isn't the natural way of speaking. Of course, 'closed questions' can limit the response to 'yes or no' but pauses and silence can allow people to expand on their thoughts. We can have 'rules' of communication and listening skills but this can mean we are not behaving naturally or comfortably, which would have a more negative impact than using the rules of active listening as an instruction manual approach. Demonstrating empathy, warmth and genuine interest is vital in any conversation of this nature, as people will feel more comfortable opening up to you if this is their perception. There are several points in the conversation above where your character helps Jessie reflect; from this, she makes decisions about how she wants to move forward. This is a brief example of an initial conversation to get to know Jessie as a person and start building a therapeutic relationship, but the same principles can be applied to more complex or distressing conversations.

Key points to consider for effective listening and communication:

- Think about the environment. If it is loud or other people are around, this is a significant barrier to effective communication. Find a quiet space where you can give someone your undivided attention
- Body Language matters. Think about how you are sitting or standing. Be mindful of fidgeting, crossing your arms or facing away from someone as this can make them feel that you don't want to be there or aren't paying attention
- Listen. It can be hard during long conversations to give someone 100% of your attention, particularly when you know you have lots of tasks to complete later but focussing on someone and what they're saying is incredibly important. Don't think about how you are going to respond while they are talking, you can take a pause when they are finished if you need to gather your thoughts
- Be mindful of your tone. We can unintentionally come across differently than we intend because of the tone we use.
- Say what you mean. We can sometimes talk in euphemisms or not be accurate with our words ('I'll be with you in one minute!' then disappearing for 20 minutes is a fairly classic example in nursing!). Sometimes, we don't know the answer, and that's ok, be honest about that and be realistic in your timeframes.
- Document carefully. Written documentation is vital in healthcare, and we sometimes forget that our notes or documentation may be needed by other teams down the line. Being clear and detailed is important as is being 100% accurate. Avoid using subjective terminology that may mean different things to different people. 'They were alright' is an example of this; if you change the tone in your mind, it can mean that they were ok, a bit off, sad, happy, etc., so use clear and professional terminology that clinicians in the future will understand.
- Eye contact is not the same for everyone. Eye contact can be difficult or uncomfortable for many, which may be very personal to them or a cultural norm. We make significant judgements in mental health based on eye contact and need to be mindful that we understand the reasons behind eye contact or a lack thereof.

Listening and communication skills are fundamental to everything we do in health and social care. We can always be honing and improving these skills but to do that, we need to be reflective and critical of our interactions. Sometimes, we don't communicate as effectively as we would have liked, but taking the time to consider these instances and learn from them is crucial to improving and developing our skills to build better therapeutic and professional relationships and improve our sense of self and wellbeing.

References

Baghbanzadeh, A., and Sobhi, A. (2021) 'A single-center cross-sectional study on the relationship between mental health, communication skills, and maladaptive schemas with nurses' job motivation'. *Chronic Diseases Journal*, 9(1), pp. 22–29. doi:10.22122/cdj.v9i1.587.

Aadam, B., Poon, A.W. and Fernandez, E. (2023) 'Listening in mental health clinical practice'. *British Journal of Social Work*, 54(1). doi:10.1093/bjsw/bcad193.

Bramhall, E. (2014) 'Effective communication skills in nursing practice'. *Nursing Standard*, 29(14), pp. 53–59. doi:10.7748/ns.29.14.53.e9355.

Fitzgerald, D.T. (2020) 'Using online active listening to facilitate student communication skills'. *Journal of Nursing Education*, 59(2), pp. 117–117. doi:10.3928/01484834-20200122-13.

Papageorgiou, A., Loke, Y.K. and Fromage, M. (2017) 'Communication skills training for mental health professionals working with people with severe mental illness'. *Cochrane Database of Systematic Reviews*, 6(6). doi:10.1002/14651858.cd010006.pub2.

Pidano, A.E., Padukkavidana, M.M. and Honigfeld, L. (2017) '"Doctor, are you listening?" Communication about children's mental health and psychosocial concerns'. *Families, Systems & Health*, 35(1), pp. 91–93. doi:10.1037/fsh0000243.

Rønning, S.B. and Bjørkly, S. (2019) 'The use of clinical role-play and reflection in learning therapeutic communication skills in mental health education: An integrative review'. *Advances in Medical Education and Practice*, 10(10), pp. 415–425. doi:10.2147/amep.s202115.

Wissow, L., Gadomski, A., Roter, D., Larson, S., Lewis, B. and Brown, J. (2011) 'Aspects of mental health communication skills training that predict parent and child outcomes in pediatric primary care'. *Patient Education and Counseling*, 82(2), pp. 226–232. doi:10.1016/j.pec.2010.03.019.

CHAPTER 6

Working with Trauma

As mental health professionals, we are inevitably surrounded by trauma in various guises that can take a significant toll on our well-being. It could be argued that our entire profession is built on supporting people who have previously or are currently experiencing trauma. Trauma is generally understood as a concept that involves an experience that is beyond the normal human realm of experience and is of a potentially life-threatening or life-limiting nature. We generally understand assaults, attacks, war, terrorist incidents, etc. to all be examples of traumatic events that could elicit psychological trauma (Clarke, 2008), but trauma can take many forms and can also include child abuse or neglect, or an accident but trauma can be much more pervasive and complex as well. Trauma can come from witnessing the distress of another, being unable to prevent an incident from occurring or bullying. Many adults carry trauma with them in some guise; it may be from something a long time ago that they almost don't recognise as 'trauma' or it may be something they don't fully acknowledge as a traumatic experience. Ultimately, anything that has a significant negative effect on us could be traumatising. Mental health nurses (and the nursing team including health care assistants, Support Workers, Nurse Associates, etc.) are the largest occupational group within mental health services and experience the highest levels of physical and verbal violence and aggression (Wilson et al. 2020) which is why we need to consider the impact of this on the nursing workforce in particular and how we can recognise the effect of working with traumatised clients and witnessing traumatic incidents not only on ourselves but also on our colleagues.

The link between childhood experiences of trauma or 'adverse childhood experiences' (ACEs) and mental health is well established and researched, with it being estimated that 47% of adults have experienced one ACE and 9% have experienced four or more ACEs (De Bellis and Zisk, 2014), which is believed to be the threshold where an individual is likely to develop a mental health issue due to those experiences. Up to 94% of adult individuals seeking mental health care or support are believed to have experienced trauma in one capacity or another (Mott and Martin, 2019) and childhood abuse is believed to be the leading factor for adults

Thriving in Mental Health Nursing, First Edition. Laura Duncan.
© 2025 John Wiley & Sons Ltd. Published 2025 by John Wiley & Sons Ltd.

seeking mental health treatment (Clarke, 2008), which further demonstrates the undeniable link between trauma and experiencing mental health issues. We must also consider that being admitted to an inpatient mental health unit, particularly against your wishes, is a traumatising experience in itself (Wilson et al. 2020) and that can also happen to individuals at a very young age. When we consider that almost half the population have experienced one ACE, this not only applies to our client group but to the staff also. This could mean that a staff member who has experienced previous ACEs or trauma as an adult may feel more or less resilient. Instances, where that specific trauma arises, may be very challenging for that individual and may mean they are unable to engage with certain incidents.

Understanding the effects of trauma on mental health is important because of the negative impact it can have on not only our clients but also ourselves as professionals. Mental health professionals are exposed to trauma in many ways in their professional lives including first-hand traumatising experiences such as witnessing self-injurious behaviours, suicide attempts or violence and aggression that may be targeted at ourselves or others but also through vicarious traumatisation. There are many different terms used interchangeably in the literature for vicarious traumatisation including 'secondary traumatic stress' and it is also frequently intertwined with burnout and compassion fatigue (Collins and Long, 2003) however I would propose that vicarious traumatisation can lead to/contribute to burnout and compassion fatigue but they are not the same phenomenon. Secondary traumatic stress is ultimately the presence of post-traumatic stress disorder (PTSD) symptoms in clinicians and is generally seen as more significant and severe than vicarious traumatisation. It is linked to a significantly increased likelihood of leaving the profession, and there is a strong correlation with having large caseloads and long working hours (Collins and Long, 2003). Burnout and compassion (including compassion fatigue) are discussed in greater depth in other chapters, but many of the 'symptoms' of burnout are similar to vicarious traumatisation, including (but not limited to) hypervigilance, irritability, anxiety, low mood and difficulties with interpersonal relationships. Hypervigilance is a response to what is ultimately perceived as a 'dangerous' environment and includes having a heightened awareness of your surroundings, being restless and agitated and appears to be present in almost all mental health professionals who have experienced violence in the workplace (Forté et al., 2017). Hypervigilance can make it particularly challenging for professionals to relax and rest effectively as most individuals continue to display hypervigilance in their personal lives. I know many mental health nurses (myself included) who still feel uncomfortable with their back to a door in a room. This is frequently joked about but is actually a symptom of ongoing hypervigilance or traumatisation, mainly when this exists many years after leaving inpatient services, where it is a legitimate safety strategy to ensure you are aware of and can see your route of exit at all times. Hypervigilance can appear very much like the 'fight or flight' response, where the individual is always ready and prepared to take action. However, this is not a psychologically or physically healthy state of being and creates significant emotional and physical stress.

Vicarious traumatisation can occur when an individual recalls and discusses or discloses a traumatic event. Practitioners are therefore exposed to vivid imagery which is ultimately, indirect exposure that can have a significant emotional impact on the practitioner (Mott and Martin, 2019). When we consider how our daily practice as mental health professionals is talking to people about their experiences, what is upsetting them and/or why they feel they may need some support; it becomes clear how frequently we may be exposed to clients discussing their traumatic experiences, commonly in great and graphic detail and therefore, how frequently we are exposed to vicarious traumatisation. Within the literature, vicarious traumatisation seems almost inevitable for clinicians who work empathetically with traumatised clients (Collins and Long, 2003). The fact that we may be exposed to trauma and vicarious trauma, however, does not dictate how we are affected or impacted by it.

Some of the impacts of indirect exposure to trauma include burnout, compassion fatigue, vicarious traumatisation and inability to engage empathetically with clients (Mott and Martin, 2019). There are a number of signs and symptoms that a clinician is experiencing vicarious traumatisation or secondary traumatic stress. Many of these symptoms are similar to the diagnostic guidelines of PTSD, including distressing emotions, depression, anxiety, extreme fear, rage, shame and strong imagery of the trauma, including nightmares and intrusive images. Individuals experiencing vicarious traumatisation may begin avoiding potential triggers, have sleep disturbances or even experience gastrointestinal issues as a somatic presentation of stress. Other signs may include addiction or compulsive behaviours that could present as being a 'workaholic', hypervigilance or what may present as poor work performance, such as missing appointments or being persistently late; however, this could be linked to general social impairment caused by traumatisation (Collins and Long, 2003). Research has shown that clinicians working in inpatient environments may start avoiding clients, become less empathetic and could even be abrasive or flippant towards clients which are indicators of experiencing vicarious traumatisation or burnout (Clarke, 2008). Research into the long-term physiological effects of trauma include an increased likelihood of developing COPD, cardiovascular disease and even an increased prevalence of autoimmune diseases, the main reason this is believed to be the case is that there is an increased likelihood of health-harming or high-risk behaviours such as smoking, excessive alcohol intake, illicit substance use, etc. (Wilson et al. 2020).

There are a number of factors that can increase an Individual's risk of being negatively affected by vicarious traumatisation and these include; general well-being, lack of social support, lack of self-care, personal history of trauma and difficulty in maintaining appropriate professional boundaries (Mott and Martin, 2019). When we consider these factors further, it would seem logical that someone who is generally emotionally and physically healthy will be in a better position to manage difficult incidents or situations than someone who is already struggling with poor physical or emotional health. Similarly, having a good support network is crucial to our general well-being and feeling able to speak to someone about a difficult incident can help us to process this in a healthy way. Individuals with higher levels of self-care are generally seen to have lower incidences of burnout, compassion fatigue and vicarious traumatisation. This is why self-care and managing our own well-being are crucial to thriving as a mental health professional and are discussed in greater depth in the 'self-care and well-being' chapter. Not all experiences of working with trauma are negative and some clinicians can experience positive effects from working with traumatised clients with some clinicians experiencing an improved sense of self and others (Collins and Long, 2003) which may be linked to their outlook on life, attitude and personal resilience. Having a positive attitude generally and considering yourself to be 'lucky' or grateful for not having the same negative experiences could seem unempathetic or even callous, but it could help not only protect our own well-being when working with trauma but also help us work with our clients in a hopeful and optimistic manner.

'Trauma-informed care' (TIC) is not a new concept in mental health; however, many clinicians feel they lack the training and resources to provide TIC, but this may be due to there being a lack of uniformity around the core principles of TIC (Wilson et al. 2020). Most can agree that the therapeutic relationship is at the heart of any TIC and an effective, person-centred recovery-focused approach (Wilson, Hutchinson and Hurley, 2017) is crucial in supporting individuals who have experienced trauma. TIC enhances the therapeutic relationship and, in particular, enhances a sensitive and compassionate consideration of an individual's behaviour rather than attaching stigmatising labels to said behaviour (Wilson et al. 2020). Many clinicians want to work in a more TIC manner and express high levels of interest in learning more about TIC, specifically to help them improve confidence in responding to disclosures of trauma and understanding the broader impact of trauma on individuals.

Activities

So how can we work in a trauma-informed way with clients? Let's explore this via a vignette:

A 45-year-old female attended her general practitioner (GP) after experiencing very distressing night terrors and reported feeling very anxious and 'panicked' throughout the day. She felt unable to relax as was terrified of going to sleep due to the nightmares she had been experiencing. Her GP was concerned with the sudden onset of symptoms and advised her to attend Accident and Emergency (A&E) to see the Psychiatric Liaison Team. Upon assessment, they feel she would benefit from an admission and assessment within an inpatient mental health facility and she consented to this, then being admitted on a voluntary basis. She had no previous history of mental health issues and had never had contact with any mental health services.

There is limited detail thus far but this was the handover I received upon admission and leads us to some important considerations:

- Initial thoughts – this is an unusual presentation. Most people who experience significant mental health issues develop symptoms in adolescence; she is 45 years of age and has never previously experienced mental health issues, which is of note.
- She is not currently pregnant, has not had a child in the past 18 months and is not yet menopausal – which are all also potential trigger periods for mental health issues.
- What these considerations lead us to is that she may have experienced a significant trauma.

Our next consideration should be how to develop a greater understanding of her symptoms and needs:

- Consider how to develop a rapport and therapeutic relationship. A therapeutic relationship should be based on genuineness and trust. This will look different to each professional but I approached her to offer her tea/coffee and asked if she would sit with me in a quiet space to discuss how we as a team could move forward in helping her
- After we feel we have developed a rapport and started our therapeutic relationship, we can approach why she presented to the GP. Examples of how we could frame these questions include;
  - What has been bothering you?
  - How does that make you feel?
  - Is there anything else on your mind?
  - How do you feel we can help you?

After spending time with her and understanding that she had been experiencing terrifying nightmares where she had the sensation of being 'pushed down' and 'held down', I allowed her the time to express these feelings. It is important within our therapeutic relationships to allow time and space for people to express their thoughts and feelings in their own time and comfort zone. Many people fear disclosing traumatic incidents as they worry, that they may not be believed or that the person they are disclosing it to will think it 'silly' or 'unimportant'. To support someone whilst discussing something traumatising, as the experience of the nightmare itself was, we can use supportive language such as the following:

- That must be really difficult.
- I'm so sorry you have experienced that.
- This would upset anyone who experienced it.
- It's a really positive step for you to tell me this so I know how to help you move forward.
- You don't always have to feel like this, there is help available.

After she had discussed the experience of the nightmares and how these had caused her to feel anxious and panicked throughout the day, as she was now frightened of going to sleep, we began to discuss what may have caused the nightmares. She reported that she had had a stressful few months with her work, but most significantly, she had experienced a family bereavement. She was able to identify that the nightmares had started at a similar time and she was able to identify that going through a very stressful period may have been what triggered the nightmares. When reflecting on how specific the nightmares were, that it was always that she was being held down or pushed, she was able to disclose that she had been the victim of an assault in her 20s where she had been held down.

Being able to understand that her recent stressful life events may have triggered previous trauma, the assault, was a significant step forward for her. She had never sought support following the assault, and she agreed that talking therapies would be a positive way forward for her as she clearly needed to work through both her historic trauma and her recent stressful events. She was able to see that there was help available and that with some support, she would recover from this episode well. She began engaging in counselling and made a quick recovery.

Within this vignette, we can see a client who has experienced significant trauma and that this is manifesting in a very challenging way for them. The key points within this vignette that help us understand how to work with clients who have experienced trauma are:

- Always give time – if someone has experienced a trauma, we need to give them space to discuss this in their own time. This may be months of working with a client before they feel able and

comfortable to disclose trauma to us but we must never rush this. In the moment of someone discussing a difficult topic, we must be patient.
- Validate – we may not feel that we would have been negatively affected by the incident/situation but this has clearly had a negative impact on them. Reinforce that it is positive they have disclosed this and that there is help available.
- Reflect – use active listening skills to ensure you have understood what they have told you correctly and support them in reflecting on how the incident has affected them. Positively reflecting on their resilience to leave a bad situation or to be brave enough to ask for help is very important
- Safeguard – if someone is the victim of abuse, we need to ensure they are appropriately safeguarded. If a crime is disclosed, we have a duty to report it so consider the immediate safety of the individual, children or others involved and escalate to your line manager or safeguarding lead if you are unsure.
- Close the wound – talking about a traumatic event, even if historic, can feel like 'opening the wound' and can cause significant distress. As professionals, our role is to allow the individual to be distressed, give them the time to express their feelings and then to 'close the wound'. This can take many different formats or approaches but helping the individual to orientate on the future by talking about their plans or goals can be a good way to do this. Before ending a session, we should 'check-in' with our clients to see how they are feeling and ensure that they are feeling ok and are able to keep themselves safe.
- Plan – ensure the client knows what will happen next. This could be 'I'm going to make you a coffee and then there will be a ward activity', 'I'll see you tomorrow' or 'I'm going to refer you to our team psychologist' but ensure that you are clear with what the next steps to support them will be.

The first vignette explored how to support clients experiencing a traumatic event; in the second vignette, we will think about how to support colleagues after a traumatic incident.

About 2 months after I first qualified as a nurse, I witnessed an incident that was, to be blunt, horrifying. It is, to this day, the most traumatic incident I have ever experienced. I will not go into details of the incident itself as that is not the focus of this vignette but it involved significant self-injurious behaviour. As with any significant incident, the safety of the client was the initial focus. He was cared for and left the unit to receive specialist, surgical intervention. Once his safety was ensured, the post-incident process began.

The incident occurred at 8 p.m., right at the end of the shift and after the incident itself was concluded, the senior nurse on shift led a debrief. No staff were injured, the incident had been managed in the best way it could have been, the service user was safe and members of the response team reported that they were a little shocked but were ok to go home. That left four of us as the ward team who had been working with the client all day.

Reflecting on the immediate period after the incident, I can now recognise that I was in shock. I vividly remember cleaning the clinic room over and over again until one of the night shift team (who was also a dear friend I had worked with for many years) came and told me to stop. I remember the overwhelming need to 'be doing something productive'. The other members of my team seemed to be experiencing the same as it was after midnight when the night staff gently ushered us all out. We documented so thoroughly that the Trust did not open a 'serious untoward incident' investigation as they felt there was no further information that could be provided.

The four of us left together; we had spent hours de-briefing and ensuring everything that could be done had been but we were all in shock. Two of us usually walked home and two drove, so we paired off and made sure we all got home safely. The next day, all of us were on days off, but we all called each other to 'check in'. When we were next on shift together, we 'checked in' again. Our line managers and supervisors held additional supervision with us all. One of the things that I remember talking about with my team and supervisors was that I kept wanting to check on the client (who was recuperating from surgery in a general hospital), even though I knew he was under the supervision of colleagues and the care of the post-surgical team. We were also getting regular feedback on how he was doing so I recognised that this was excessive and didn't act on it, but that feeling wouldn't leave me until he returned to the mental health unit. When that happened, he was admitted to a different ward and I asked permission to go and see him. He was doing ok, his mental state was vastly improved, and physically, he would have no lasting damage, which was wonderful news. I vividly remember the feeling of relief at seeing that he was 'ok'.

Even today, when I reflect on this incident that happened over a decade ago, I feel guilty. I have intrusive images of the incident itself but the overwhelming thought of 'we should have seen it coming' is the most distressing. We didn't see it coming and that was the core focus of all of our reflections in the aftermath, picking apart the hours before the incident in minute detail. Logically, I know that there were no obvious precipitants. All four of us had engaged with him throughout the day; he had seemed calm, his partner had visited him, there was no history of this type of behaviour or level of distress and so there was nothing that could have predicted what was to happen. However, logic and emotions are very different. Sometimes, we will never fully rationalise our thoughts and emotions about something but I can use my reflective skills to understand that we did all we could.

There will be distressing incidents in the career of any mental health professional. Hopefully, they will not be as distressing as this example, but we do need to accept that we will be witnessing things that are traumatising in nature. While nothing can erase that it happened, we can ensure that we support ourselves and our colleagues when difficult incidents do happen.

The key messages from this vignette are as follows:

- Debrief immediately – ensure everyone is safe and there are no injuries. Ask people their feelings and be supportive if a colleague is distressed. Ensure tasks are completed like incident forms etc., but the physical and emotional safety of your team and the client is the ultimate priority.
- Acknowledge your own emotions.
- Talk to your colleagues, make sure they are ok and tell them if you are not.
- Use supervision – clinical and managerial supervision is there to support you and to develop you; learning from difficult incidents is necessary and supervision is the place to do this and express your thoughts and feelings openly.
- If an incident has caused you distress, seek help. Go to counselling, find a therapist, see your GP – do whatever you would advise others to do and tell your line manager how you are feeling.

If I had not engaged with my colleagues and team, if I had not felt supported and cared for as a colleague, this incident could have been disastrous for my personal well-being. As it was, I worked with some incredible professionals who demonstrated the highest levels of support and team working you could hope for.

References

Clarke, V. (2008) 'Working with survivors of trauma', *Mental Health Practice*, 11(7), pp. 14–17. doi:10.7748/mhp2008.04.11.7.14.c6481.

Collins, S. and Long, A. (2003) 'Working with the psychological effects of trauma: Consequences for mental health-care workers – A literature review', *Journal of Psychiatric and Mental Health Nursing*, 10(4), pp. 417–424. doi:10.1046/j.1365-2850.2003.00620.x.

De Bellis, M.D. and Zisk, A. (2014) 'The biological effects of childhood trauma', *Child and Adolescent Psychiatric Clinics of North America*, 23(2), pp. 185–222. doi:10.1016/j.chc.2014.01.002.

Forté, L. et al. (2017) 'Experiencing violence in a psychiatric setting: Generalized hypervigilance and the influence of caring in the fear experienced', *Work*, 57(1), pp. 55–67. doi:10.3233/wor-172540.

Mott, J. and Martin, L.A. (2019) 'Adverse childhood experiences, self-care, and Compassion Outcomes in mental health providers working with trauma', *Journal of Clinical Psychology*, 75(6), pp. 1066–1083. doi:10.1002/jclp.22752.

Wilson, A., Hurley, J., Hutchinson, M. and Lakeman, R. (2020). 'Can mental health nurses working in acute mental health units really be trauma-informed? An integrative review of the literature. *Journal of Psychiatric and Mental Health Nursing*, 28(5), pp.900–923. doi: doi.org/10.1111/jpm.12717.

Wilson, A., Hutchinson, M. and Hurley, J. (2017) 'Literature review of trauma-informed care: Implications for mental health nurses working in acute inpatient settings in Australia', *International Journal of Mental Health Nursing*, 26(4), pp. 326–343. doi:10.1111/inm.12344.

CHAPTER 7

Working with Risk

'Risk' is an everyday consideration for a Mental Health Professional (Downes et al., 2016) and can sometimes be such a focus of the clinical role that it overshadows all other aspects of assessment (Newton-Howes, 2018). Maintaining safety and managing risk has always been considered one of the 'highest profile' aspects of a mental health professional's role, particularly nurses (Higgins et al., 2015). One of the consequences of risk being seen to be so 'high profile' in Mental Health Services is that completing risk assessments can become very anxiety-provoking for clinicians as the concern about potentially being wrong and what that could mean can be very concerning (Gale et al., 2016).

It may be a central concept within mental health practice, but what do we actually mean by 'risk'? The basis of any consideration of risk and its meaning is a negative outcome that is yet uncertain (Nathan, Whyler and Wilson, 2020) and trying to understand risk is about trying to ascertain the likelihood of a certain outcome (Newton-Howes, 2018). Risk is generally associated with 'dangerousness' and danger (Downes et al., 2016), and in mental health, we tend to consider the most serious potential outcomes as our key risk areas, such as suicide or homicide; however, it is actually the much more common risks that also need to be part of everyday risk assessments such as managing an independent life and looking after yourself (Newton-Howes, 2018) that also need to be considered. Forensic Mental Health services have a very strong focus on risk, most commonly risk of violence towards others, however the actual evidence to support that individuals with mental health issues are more likely to be violent towards others is generally considered to be weak, and so even in higher security services, the concerns regarding violence or committing criminal offences must also be balanced with recovery focussed care (O'Dowd, Cohen and Quayle, 2022). There are many types of risk that are frequently overlooked that do pose a significant concern to the individual's well-being that are under-considered, such as the risk of intimate partner violence or sexual abuse, which is believed to be a much more frequent phenomenon for those with significant mental health issues (Higgins et al., 2015). This highlights the need for holistically focussed risk assessments that take into account the individual's social

Thriving in Mental Health Nursing, First Edition. Laura Duncan.
© 2025 John Wiley & Sons Ltd. Published 2025 by John Wiley & Sons Ltd.

circumstances and the people around them. These considerations could include; 'what is their relationship status?', 'does this person feel safe at home?', 'what are the risks of worsening mood if this person is socially isolated?' or 'is there a risk of malnutrition or poor health outcomes if this individual is struggling to manage their food and fluid intake well?' and whilst these considerations do usually get considered within care planning or an Activities of Daily Living assessments, they are also risks to the person's holistic well-being and shouldn't be overshadowed by the 'worst case scenario' risks such as suicide, self-harm or violence. Where such serious risks are identified, of course, they do need to become a priority to ensure the safety of the client and others, but we shouldn't lose sight of the more holistic perspective of risk at the same time.

We hear the term 'risk aversion' frequently in the literature and in clinical practice and it is generally understood that a clinician being 'risk averse' is a person who is ultimately being protective of their client for fear of a negative outcome for them but in trying to be protective, we may not be recovery focussed and helping that client to move forward in their life. One reason that is cited frequently in the literature for mental health professionals being 'risk averse' is that there is a general public perception of 'dangerousness' that could possibly impact professionals in the sense that they are more likely to be risk-averse and engage in 'defensive' practice (O'Dowd, Cohen and Quayle, 2022) due to concerns of the public perception. Providing public reassurance has been a central feature of risk assessments as public perceptions of danger and 'dramatic risks' have been heightened following high-profile incidents and negative media representations of individuals with mental health issues (Higgins et al., 2015). The complexity of the issue is where practitioners find themselves trying to balance safety with autonomy and having to consider potential repercussions for any negative outcomes (Downes et al., 2016) which highlights the pressure an individual clinician may feel when completing a risk assessment in clinical practice.

Historically, risk assessment has been focussed on attempting to eliminate and control all risks (Downes et al., 2016), which we now understand is an impossibility. However, the literature suggests that nurses' conceptualisations of risk continue to focus on the assessment, management and prevention of all risks (Higgins et al., 2015). We must now understand that even with all factors being optimal, no risk assessment is perfect and there are consistently false positives and false negatives with any risk assessment tool (Higgins et al., 2015). This is basically due to the fact that no one can predict the future, no matter how good the assessment tool you use is! There is significant debate within the literature as to whether risk assessment tools are actually helpful at all, as they are based on group data and behaviour rather than the individual and have a tendency to err on the side of caution rather than recovery (Downes et al., 2016). As risk assessment is a core part of a mental health nurses' role, there has been the assumption that nurses are proficient in this area, however, the literature suggests that inter-rater reliability of risk assessments is often very poor (Gale et al., 2016). What this means is that two nurses could use the same risk assessment tool with the same client and have different outcomes. Many of the risk assessment tools utilised in clinical practice do not account for physical health risks, financial or sexual exploitation, victimisation or harassment (Higgins et al., 2015) which leads us to the conclusion that they are not only not necessarily reliable for high-consequence risks such as suicide, self-harm or violence but also not assessing holistically for risks that may actually be occurring more frequently. Where certain tools may be very helpful in framing a risk assessment and supporting a clinician in approaching a thorough risk assessment, most nurses believe their instinct and own assessment skills are more accurate than risk assessment tools (Downes et al., 2016) and many mental health nurses report that they rely on their instinct or intuition heavily when it comes to understanding risk (Higgins et al., 2015).

Positive risk-taking is a key concept in recovery-focussed care, and it is, therefore, a professional's role to work with risk in a proactive manner (Downes et al., 2016). Positive risk-taking focusses more on an individual's personal growth and development; there is also a move away from focusing on 'dramatic risk' and is more collaborative in nature (Higgins et al., 2015). As already discussed, assessing risk in the first place can be very complex and challenging for even the most experienced clinician, so the concept of not just trying to minimise and mitigate risk but to support a client in which risks are, on balance, 'ok' to take can be a very daunting and frightening prospect. Because of this, the multidisciplinary team (MDT) is a key factor in good quality risk assessment and management plans, as individuals who feel that the MDT communicates effectively and listens are more likely to engage in the risk assessment process in a more collaborative and effective way (O'Dowd, Cohen and Quayle, 2022). This highlights the importance of working with the team in an honest, open and transparent way. Many clinicians work in environments where they are 'lone working' with clients but good practice is to have frequent case discussions with the MDT in a supportive and collegiate manner.

Another factor that can be challenging for clinicians is how to ask those difficult questions but risk assessment and management should always be a joint endeavour between clinicians and clients. This can cause challenges for many clinicians as they can be concerned about having challenging conversations and that this could potentially damage their therapeutic relationship with the individual (O'Dowd, Cohen and Quayle, 2022). With this in mind, we are going to consider how to approach difficult questions, what happens when risk assessments go wrong and how to manage your own feelings about risk.

Activities

How to Approach Difficult Questions

The core consideration here is the clinical environment where you are practicing. In each type of service, the approach to risk assessments will be significantly different, so, you will need to consider the needs of your client group and service to apply these principles to your practice. The approach discussed here came from my clinical practice when I was working in courts and police stations as part of my role as a liaison and diversion practitioner within the criminal justice system. The core focus of my role was to complete assessments with individuals who had been arrested or were appearing in court, usually in custody, but some clients were on bail when I worked with them. This meant that I had to conduct a very rapid assessment with someone who I had (usually) never met before in a challenging environment (court/policy custody suites are not the most 'homely' places!) to establish what their health, well-being and social needs were, establish a plan with them and then report this to the police or court. Establishing a rapport quickly is a significant challenge, but in this type of role, an absolute priority. The nature and complexity of the role meant that I had a significant amount of information to gather about each individual I assessed, and this can very quickly begin to feel like an interrogation for the individual. Because of how conscious I was of this not becoming the case, I wrote my own assessment tool. This is something I recommend frequently to anyone who is conducting assessments on a regular basis. Within the construction of my assessment tool, I not only considered the information I needed to establish but also how I was going to ask the questions. I then considered how to 'cluster' the questions so that it felt more like a conversation with a natural flow rather than an interview. I would then periodically reflect on my assessments and how they had gone, were there any areas that weren't flowing well or felt jarring? If so, I would review my tool and the way I formulated my questions to try and address these areas and continue doing this throughout my time in liaison and diversion services.

To begin an assessment, we must, of course, introduce ourselves and explain our role. Below is how I would typically do this:

> 'Hi, my name is Laura and I'm a mental health nurse here at – court/police station. I wanted to meet with you to see if there's anything that's bothering your or upsetting you at the moment that I could possibly help you with, is that ok?'

Once initial consent to the assessment has been gained, I would then move on to confidentiality and liaising:

> 'Anything you say to me, I may put in a report for the court/police station, is that ok?'

Then:

> 'Are you happy for me to contact your GP or any other services you may have had contact with?'

If verbal consent is given to all, then the assessment can begin. If they have questions, then, of course, those would need to be addressed, and if someone did not consent to the assessment or information being shared with the court/police, then the assessment could not go ahead. If an individual did not want their general physician (GP) or other services to be informed, this could be discussed in terms of what their concerns were and why they may be worried about this, and these could then be addressed but if they did refuse consent to liaise with other services, then I would advise that I may not be able to refer them to services that could help but we could review this at the end of the assessment. If someone were to decline, I would politely accept and advise them that if they changed their mind and did want to speak to me, they could just ask the custody staff and they would contact me to come back.

This may seem basic; the phrasing may seem unusual or uncomfortable to you, but that is why I have included it so explicitly. This phrasing is comfortable and natural *for me*, and this is precisely the reason that we should all consider how we ask questions in an assessment.

Once consent and introductions have been completed, we can move on to the assessment itself. In structuring my assessments, I considered that most people are quite comfortable sharing/confirming their demographic data. So, in the interest of establishing rapport, this is where I would start. Ask them to confirm their name and date of birth, then their address. Once I asked for their address, this is where I began 'clustering' information to make the assessment flow more naturally.

'Can you tell me where you have been living recently if you do have an address?' This will obviously tell me if they are experiencing homelessness, which would then lead the assessment in a different direction, but if they confirm they do have a stable address, then I would ask 'Do you feel safe there?' this question allows me to start understanding whether there are any other housing issues like crime, mould, damp, etc. but gives a critical insight into their home life and whether there are issues I need to explore in more depth. The next question would be:

> 'Who do you live with there?' This question will then start to tell me about their social situation in a little more detail: do they have a partner/family/children, etc.? If they confirm they do live with others, I would then ask 'How is your relationship with them?' This question can give an insight into whether there are any relationship issues, including domestic violence, exploitation, or abuse.

As you can see in this vignette, I have asked fairly simple questions but have focussed on the person becoming more comfortable in the assessment environment and with me as the assessor. The key principle in any assessment is allowing the person to express themselves in their own words and time. If, for example, following these questions, the individual has informed me that they live with a partner but do not feel safe at home because of a violent or abusive relationship, this is obviously a very significant and serious piece of information. Instead of moving on to the next cluster of questions, I would explore this in more depth and try to establish a plan of 'next steps' with the individual, asking in particular what they would like to happen next.

Being flexible and agile in an assessment will mean you are able to garner information in a more natural way and will also identify the key areas you need to focus on more easily. In the example above, there is a very serious risk issue identified that you can then focus on to try and understand more thoroughly and plan with the client how to move forward.

When we consider the 'difficult' questions, such as those around suicide, self-harm, drug and alcohol use or psychosis; for example, we obviously must include these questions in any assessment to establish if there are any risks or issues in these areas. The approach I have always utilised is introducing the question theme to give the client some warning of what will come next and more of a sense of control of the situation:

> 'I have some difficult questions to ask you now but I have to ask everyone, is that ok?'

If they agree, I would then proceed with the questions to establish the needs in those areas, giving them time and space to express their thoughts and feelings throughout.

When formulating the level of risk, we need to consider key questions such as:

- What do I think the risk is?
- When would the risk potentially occur?
- How would it potentially occur?
- Who would likely be involved?
- Where would it potentially happen?
- How likely is this risk to occur?

If we use suicide as an example, we need to consider whether the client is experiencing suicidal thoughts, if they have any intent on acting on those thoughts, if there are any protective factors and if they have a plan.

If client 1 states:

> 'I've been having some really dark thoughts and think everyone would just be better off without me but I have friends and family who would be upset if I hurt myself so I don't think I'd ever do anything and I've never thought about how I'd do it'.

If another client states:

> 'I don't want to be here anymore, as soon as I leave here, I'm going to the nearest railway bridge and jumping in front of a train. There's nothing in my life anymore and no-one who cares'.

We can immediately see that the level of risk is very different. The first client clearly needs help and support because they don't have to feel that way, but they are unlikely to harm themselves. We can establish a plan with them of how to get them some support and give them crisis guidance and information in case they do begin to feel worse. The second client, however, is being very clear and is at very high risk of trying to end their life. This client needs a much more immediate plan to support them and would likely benefit from either intensive community support or being admitted to an inpatient unit as we can clearly see that there is a very imminent, immediate and life-threatening risk in what they have said.

What Happens When Risk Assessments Go Wrong and How Do We Manage Our Feelings?

Many clinicians can be very fearful of what may happen if they make a 'mistake', and this is not just limited to risk assessments but they are an important aspect of this fear. As professionals, we can worry about not only the consequences to the client but also the consequences to ourselves, such as disciplinary procedures or losing our professional reputation or registration. In reality, it is very rare and unusual that a clinical decision that was made in good faith would ever lead to such significant repercussions for a professional, particularly if we can evidence our decision-making and reasoning and are honest and transparent with any investigations that may occur. We can be reasonably reassured of this by our colleagues and team, but what can ultimately be much harder to reckon with is when there is a negative consequence for a client.

I think the hardest situation to process is if we have had contact with a client who then takes their own life. We may have understood the severity of the risk and may have put many protective factors in place but it can be very difficult to process those feelings. I once had a client who I immediately recognised was very likely to try and end their life if they were remanded into custody (i.e., went to prison), and so I did everything that I could and should have done in that scenario. I ensured he was on constant watch in court and that he would be assessed by the mental health team in prison, and I contacted them directly to refer him. It was very unusual for me to be as blunt as this, but my level of concern for this client was that I told them that I believed as soon as he was no longer on constant observation, that he would attempt to end his life. A month later, he took his own life in prison. I didn't actually find out about what had happened until I was contacted by The Coroners Court, which was incredibly upsetting but also terrified me as I had never had to attend Coroners Court previously. I raised it with my line manager immediately, and they were incredibly supportive, they gave me guidance and offered to help me prepare for attending court but also acknowledged that I was very sad and upset that this gentleman had passed away. I provided all of my notes, reports and correspondence about his case to The Coroners Court, and they ultimately felt that I didn't need to attend in person as my documentation had been very clear about my assessment and involvement in the case. I accessed supervision to process my feelings about the case and asked my line manager to review all of my actions to establish if there was anything else I could or should have done in that scenario when we established that my assessment had been of good quality and I had taken all the reasonable steps available to me, it did help me move forward and not question my skills or ability in similar situations in the future.

We can try our hardest to be perfect practitioners, but ultimately, we cannot predict the future, and if we are working in a recovery-focused way, sometimes we need to acknowledge there is a risk and empower the client to address this in their own way. We can rationalise all of this, but we are still human beings with feelings. It can be terrifying to allow a risk to continue to be a risk rather than trying to manage or eradicate it, particularly if that risk comes to fruition. This is where we need to acknowledge our own skills, be clear about our risk assessments and why we have made the decisions we have made and taken the actions we have taken, and ensure that we use supervision and support our colleagues and teams when risks or negative outcomes do occur.

References

Downes, C. et al. (2016) 'Survey of mental health nurses' attitudes towards risk assessment, risk assessment tools and positive risk', *Journal of Psychiatric and Mental Health Nursing*, 23(3–4), pp. 188–197. doi:10.1111/jpm.12299.

Gale, T.M. et al. (2016) 'Perception of suicide risk in mental health professionals', *PLoS One*, 11(2). doi:10.1371/journal.pone.0149791.

Higgins, A. et al. (2015) 'There is more to risk and safety planning than dramatic risks: Mental Health Nurses' risk assessment and safety-management practice', *International Journal of Mental Health Nursing*, 25(2), pp. 159–170. doi:10.1111/inm.12180.

Nathan, R., Whyler, J. and Wilson, P. (2020) 'Risk of harm to others: Subjectivity and meaning of risk in mental health practice', *Journal of Risk Research*, 24(10), pp. 1228–1238. doi:10.1080/13669877.2020.1819389.

Newton-Howes, G. (2018) 'Risk in mental health: A review on and of the psychiatrist', *The Journal of Mental Health Training, Education and Practice*, 13(1), pp. 14–21. doi:10.1108/jmhtep-04-2017-0030.

O'Dowd, R., Cohen, M.H. and Quayle, E. (2022) 'A systematic mixed studies review and framework synthesis of mental health professionals' experiences of violence risk assessment and management in Forensic Mental Health Settings', *Journal of Forensic Psychology Research and Practice*, 23(1), pp. 21–55. doi:10.1080/24732850.2021.2013364.

CHAPTER 8

Diversity and Inclusivity

Respect for diversity and inclusivity has gained increasing prominence across all aspects of modern life, but many may not fully appreciate its importance, what it means as a concept, its impact when not upheld or its relevance to health and mental health. In short, 'inclusivity' is when people from all communities and backgrounds feel welcome, respected and able to be themselves (Lane, 2021). When people feel excluded or unable to be their true authentic selves, there can be a significant impact on their health and well-being. 'Diversity' is about understanding that people are different, have different experiences and live unique lives. Diversity is usually divided into 'social' and 'cultural', but it can be hard to specify which particular focus each aspect, such as religion, gender, ethnicity, sexual orientation, etc. would fall under as many tend to impact both our social and cultural understanding of the world. As health and social care professionals, we have a duty to have an awareness of both cultural and social diversity as well as promote social justice (Kung and Johansson, 2022) to address and tackle inequality, stigma and discrimination when we are aware of it. At the core of ethical practice as a clinician is maintaining dignity and understanding diversity and inclusivity needs is crucial to ensuring dignity is maintained and upheld (Kung and Johansson, 2022). When someone's diversity needs are not met, and they are excluded, this would usually be considered to be discrimination. Ultimately, experiencing discrimination of any kind is a significant stressor that can negatively impact well-being and mental health (Sutter and Perrin, 2016), and any group that is marginalised or in the minority in society, may experience stigma and discrimination. This highlights why it is crucial for mental health professionals, in particular, to understand the experience of individuals who are much more likely to experience discrimination due to their ethnicity, race, mental health needs, gender or sexuality. Those who experience multiple forms of discrimination, such as racism, homophobia or misogyny, are at significantly increased risk of developing mental health issues (Williams and Etkins, 2021). So, we must develop our knowledge and skills in all areas of cultural competence to ensure we are supporting people effectively and treating everyone with dignity and respect.

Thriving in Mental Health Nursing, First Edition. Laura Duncan.
© 2025 John Wiley & Sons Ltd. Published 2025 by John Wiley & Sons Ltd.

The Equality Act (2010) is a key legislation that ensures that rights are protected for those who may otherwise face discrimination and persecution due to who they are or where they are from. The Equality Act (2010) provide nine 'Protected Characteristics' that make it illegal to discriminate against someone because they possess these characteristics. The nine Protected Characteristics are:

- Age
- Disability
- Gender Reassignment
- Marriage and Civil Partnership
- Pregnancy and Maternity
- Race
- Religion or Belief
- Sex
- Sexual Orientation

All characteristics are, of course, important but certain groups within this face specific issues when it comes to health and mental health, which this chapter will have a more detailed focus on. For example, 'marriage and civil partnership' does not appear to cause mental health issues specifically, there are, of course, considerations, such as domestic violence, which would have an impact on mental health and well-being but this is not due to being discriminated against due to marital status. 'Pregnancy and maternity' have special consideration in mental health as Perinatal mental health services evidence, and there are specific mental health needs during pregnancy and the post-partum period, but again, discrimination is not the critical issue for this.

Perceived discrimination of any nature has a negative impact on well-being (Vogt Yuan, 2007) and within healthcare, we have age boundaries for certain types of services, such as Mental Health Services where we commonly have Child and Adolescent Mental Health Services (CAMHS) that support clients up to the age of 18, 'working-age adult' services that support clients between 18 and 65 years old and 'older adult' services that provide specific support to clients over 65. These age boundaries are helpful in some ways but binary, is there a significant difference in terms of need for someone aged 64 vs. someone aged 66? For older adults, there are multiple factors that can impact their mental health negatively including bereavement, loneliness and physical health issues which can lead to depression and even suicidal ideation (Aharon, Aisenberg-Shafran and Levi-Belz, 2023). However, many of our older adult services focus on Dementia as a condition specifically, which means that other clinical needs, such as depression, may be overlooked or unsupported. We see ageism within healthcare services and this can manifest as an unwillingness to provide care for older adults, more negative attitudes towards recovery and that poor mental health is perceived as 'normal' (Aharon, Aisenberg-Shafran and Levi-Belz, 2023). There can be both positive and negative stereotypes associated with ageing such as seeing older adults as warm and kind but also as less capable than working-age adults (Vogt Yuan, 2007). As clinicians, we need to ensure that we are working holistically and in a recovery-focussed way for anyone, regardless of age.

The term 'disability' includes any condition that causes challenges to engaging in activities or navigating the environment and these can be physiological or psychological conditions (Namkung and Carr, 2020). Stigma and discrimination and their impact in relation to mental health conditions are covered extensively in the 'stigma and discrimination' chapter and so here we will focus on the impact of physical disabilities on mental health. 'Ableism' is the term used for discrimination against those with disabilities and is commonly seen as a lack of thought, planning or preparation to support those with disabilities to be able to engage with the environment comfortably and would include examples such as not including appropriate ramps for wheelchair users meaning they cannot access certain places. Ableism creates inequalities and can impact all areas of life including employment, education and housing (Brown and Ciciurkaite, 2022). Without appropriate support, adjustments or adaptations, individuals with a disability may have significant difficulties in engaging in activities they would like to (or need to) and this can cause increased rates of depression or generally poorer life satisfaction (Namkung and Carr, 2020). Those who experience disability are believed to have increased rates of depression, and this is considered to be due to higher rates of social stressors (Brown and Ciciurkaite, 2022). Stressors can be further caused by experiencing the 'primary stressor' of having a disability as this can lead to financial insecurity, experience of discrimination or social exclusion (Namkung and Carr, 2020). Disabilities are highly varied and can include mobility, vision, hearing, intellectual ability, mental health needs or physical health conditions that cause pain as a few examples (this is by no means exhaustive, though). As mental health professionals, we must consider the impact of experiencing any disability, the impact of pain, ableism and accessibility of services and care to ensure we are not excluding individuals from receiving appropriate care and treatment but are also acknowledging the additional daily stressors that someone with a disability may experience.

Racism has long been understood to be a significant determinant of health; however, the detrimental impact of systemic and individual experiences of racism on mental health specifically are lesser understood and researched (Desai et al., 2023). Racism has been described as a 'public health crisis' that has a significant negative impact on young people that can persevere through adult life, with those experiencing racial discrimination at the age of 13 having a significant increase of depressive symptoms by the age of 14 (Simon, 2023). Experiencing racism during adolescence is strongly associated with a higher risk of not only anxiety and depression but also lower self-esteem, emotional regulation issues and suicidality (Bernard et al., 2020). The impact of racism can become generational where the parent's experience of racism can have a negative impact directly on their children, and this can be due to racism having an impact on the parent's mental health, their parenting behaviour or both (Simela et al., 2024). The impact of racism on young people is believed to heighten the effect and impact of other, non-racism based stress and traumas, with those from Black, Asian, minority and ethnic backgrounds being more likely to report multiple adverse childhood experiences (ACEs) than those from a White ethnic backgrounds (Bernard et al., 2020). Overt and subtle racism (also known as macro- and micro-aggressions) contribute to both long- and short-term mental health and physical health issues (Bernard et al., 2020). Racism permeates all social and institutional systems and is not limited to individual beliefs or behaviours (Williams and Etkins, 2021), and this, unfortunately, includes healthcare services. Micro-aggressions are subtle and often unintentional discriminatory words or actions; however, they can have a significant impact on the person experiencing the microaggression (Lane, 2021). In one study, up to 82% of individuals reported experiencing microaggressions whilst engaging in therapy sessions (Kung and Johansson, 2022). Research has also found that those from Black backgrounds are more likely to be diagnosed with psychotic disorders than their White counterparts when reporting the same symptoms (Williams and Etkins, 2021). The diagnostic manuals have attempted to address the issue of misdiagnosis due to cultural differences by advising clinicians to recognise that behavioural traits such as eye contact and body language vary significantly across cultures and should not be pathologized if culturally normative (Kung and Johansson, 2022). Within educational systems, although diversity has improved in terms of access to higher education for individuals from Black, Asian, minority and ethnic backgrounds, there continues to be concerning levels of racism across institutions including micro and macro aggressions such as asking students of colour to represent their entire race in discussions as well as overtly racist behaviours and discriminatory language (Kruse, Rakha and Calderon, 2017). This highlights that although many believe that racism has improved in fields such as healthcare and education, there are still significant and ongoing issues that need addressing to ensure inclusivity.

There has been a concerning rise in religious discrimination and violence or hate crimes being perpetrated against individuals because of their perceived religion (Scheitle, Frost and Ecklund, 2023). Discrimination can cause distress and negative emotions as it may cause the individual to feel that their well-being has been threatened in one capacity or another due to the perceived discrimination (Wu and Schimmele, 2019). It is important to note that the term 'perceived discrimination' is not intended to dilute the experience, it is actually about highlighting that it is the person who has experienced the discrimination who determines whether it is discrimination or not, not the perpetrator of the discrimination in terms of their intent. The potential for negative emotions due to the concern of potential harm is of course valid for all forms of discrimination but in recent years, particularly post post-Brexit referendum in the UK, there has been a significant increase in racist or religious-based hate crimes (Williams et al., 2022). Religious discrimination is higher amongst religious minorities but can be experienced by any religious group (Wu and Schimmele 2019). It is believed that those from Muslim or Jewish backgrounds in particular have experienced a significant rise in religious discrimination (Scheitle, Frost and Ecklund, Scheitle et al. 2023) and this is referred to as 'Islamophobia' and 'antisemitism', respectively. In terms of understanding the population data about religion, The ONS (Office for National Statistics, 2021) reported from the 2021 census of England and Wales that within the UK population:

- 46.2% identify as Christian,
- 6.5% identify as Muslim,
- 1.7% identify as Hindu,
- 0.9% identify as Sikh,
- 0.5% identify as Jewish and
- 0.5% identify as Buddhist.

As we can see, in England and Wales, Christianity is the majority religion by a significant margin and although Christians in the UK could experience religious discrimination, it is much less likely when almost 50% of the population identify as Christian. All discrimination is potentially harmful to health (Schietle, Frost and Ecklund, 2023) due to the impact of stress on our physical health and well-being, and so it must be acknowledged and understood. The research regarding religious discrimination however is inconsistent and ultimately inconclusive as to how significant the impact of religious discrimination is on health and the potential explanation for this is that belonging to a community that is empathetic to the experience of discrimination, may act as a 'buffer' to the negative impact of discrimination (Scheitle, Frost and Ecklund, 2023). This highlights the impact of social support on our health and well-being as it can help us to manage very significant stressors within our lives when they occur and ultimately protect our health and well-being. Within health and social care, we must acknowledge the importance of faith, religion and spirituality for the individual and help to support them in expressing this as they choose. That could be ensuring access to religious texts, items such as prayer mats or support to observe religious events such as Shabbat or Ramadan. As professionals, we do not need to know the in-depth details of all religions, but we should be comfortable in asking individuals how we can best support them and what their needs are in a respectful way.

Discrimination and mental health based on sex is a challenging picture. Gender is a social construct (Hosang and Bhui, 2018) and so for the purpose of this discussion, we refer to 'males' and 'females' based on sex and use the binary terms of 'male and female' or 'men and women' and considerations relating to individuals who are nonbinary or Transgender are included within the discussion around the lesbian, gay, bisexual, transgender, queer/questioning, plus (others) (LGBTQ+) community below. Some research suggests mental health issues affect men and women equally; however, women are more exposed to gender-based discrimination in the form of lower paying or responsibility jobs, lower social status and challenges with accessing healthcare (Hosang and Bhui, 2018). Gender discrimination is associated with lower self-esteem in women (Kucharska, 2017) and women who do not conform to societal norms can face stigma as well as social exclusion or even violence (Hosang and Bhui, 2018). Over 50% of women report experiencing sexual harassment in the workplace in the UK (Hosang and Bhui, 2018) which can have a significant impact not only in terms of the distress the incident/incidents may cause but the stress of whether to report the experience or not and how it would be managed or resolved. It would also impact how the individual feels about the workplace and whether they feel safe or comfortable to continue working there, therefore having a significant impact on employment security. In terms of the difference between the sexes from a mental health perspective, men are three times as likely as women to die by suicide and males aged 40–49 years have the highest suicide rates in the UK (Mental Health Foundation, 2022). Women are more frequently diagnosed with mood and anxiety disorders (Kucharska, 2017), which seems to conflict with the male suicide prevalence as we believe that those experiencing depression most commonly will attempt to end their lives. Perceived gender discrimination has been associated with an increase in mental health issues, including depression and post-traumatic stress disorder (PTSD) (Hosang and Bhui, 2018). Women are 3 times more likely to experience common mental health issues, eating disorders or PTSD (Mental Health Foundation, 2022). From these considerations, we can see that the gender-based picture in terms of mental health is complex. It could be suggested that women are more likely to seek help earlier which would potentially explain the higher diagnostic rates for conditions such as anxiety and depression but also the higher suicide rates for males if they are not seeking help or support. The higher prevalence of Eating Disorders could be linked to gender discrimination in the sense that it has been significantly correlated with lower self-esteem, but there is also a socially more significant focus on what is 'beauty' in terms of the female body and so this would likely play a significant role as well. In terms of our role as mental health professionals, it is important to understand the gender differences and the gender discrimination that women, in particular, may face so that we can support both males and females appropriately and fairly.

LGBTQ+ is a community of individuals who identify as lesbian, gay, bisexual, transgender, queer/questioning, intersex, asexual, nonbinary and ultimately anyone who doesn't identify as heterosexual, heteroromantic (having romantic feelings for the opposite gender) and cisgender (identifying as the gender you were born as) with the '+' being the ultimate signal of inclusivity as it is recognised that sometimes people may not feel that they 'fit' into a specific identity and that is ok and accepted. Although there has been some progress in improving equality for the LGBTQ+ community, stigma and discrimination are still prevalent (Bailey et al., 2022) with those from the LGBTQ+ community being more likely to experience violence, stigma and discrimination than those who identify as heterosexual and cisgender (Whaibeh et al. 2019). It has also been found that particularly for older members of the LGBTQ+ community, health outcomes are poorer (Bailey et al., 2022). Those from the LGBTQ+ community are more likely to experience discrimination in the workplace which is strongly correlated with poorer physical, social and mental health outcomes (Seiler-Ramadas et al., 2021). LGBTQ+ individuals have higher rates of mental health issues such as depression and anxiety (Bailey et al., 2022). Young people within the LGBTQ+ community are at increased risk of self-harm and suicide in comparison to their heterosexual and cisgender counterparts; however, it is important to avoid framing being a member of the LGBTQ+ community as being inherently vulnerable or victimised (Bryan and Mayock, 2016). One of the core reasons for the increased prevalence of mental health issues is believed to be 'heterosexism'. Heterosexism is the phenomenon when discrimination occurs because of the presumption of heterosexuality and this can lead to those from the LGBTQ+ community feeling the need to conceal their sexual or gender identity, which can significantly affect their well-being (Bialer and McIntosh, 2017). Feeling the need to conceal your identity is psychologically taxing and can have adverse effects on overall well-being (Sutter and Perrin, 2016). As with all 'stressors', one of the key determining factors as to the impact it will have is levels of support. Individuals from the LGBTQ+ community who felt they had experienced rejection from their family had a significantly increased risk of attempting suicide (Sutter and Perrin, 2016). Those from the Trans community face increased rates of prejudice and discrimination and some research suggests that almost 60% of Trans individuals have symptoms of depression (Sutter and Perrin, 2016). There is believed to be a lack of cultural competence from clinicians due to a lack of training in the specific needs of the LGBTQ+ community (Whaibeh, et al., 2019) and this leads to Trans individuals having negative experiences in care settings including being deliberately and intentionally misgendered and experiencing hostility from care workers (Bailey et al., 2022). Intentional misgendering is never acceptable and is the antithesis of treating someone with respect and dignity. We must remember that feeling accepted by family and social connections has a significant impact on the mental health of those from the LGBTQ+ community (Whaibeh, et al., 2019) and this extends to our role as healthcare professionals. We must demonstrate respect and dignity for all and ensure that those in our care feel accepted and supported to be their true, authentic selves.

So the question becomes, as healthcare professionals, what can we do to support individuals from all backgrounds and address stigma and discrimination? The answer is to improve our 'Cultural Competence'. Being culturally competent means having insight and knowledge of an individual's culture, being emotionally attuned to a client's needs, understanding our own biases and having the ability to adjust our clinical skills and approaches accordingly (Kung and Johansson, 2022). One example of cultural competency could include understanding when someone comes from a family-centred culture and offering to involve the person's family members in discussions and plans for their care and treatment (Kung and Johansson, 2022). 'Unconscious biases' are the beliefs and stereotypes that we hold that we may not be aware of or recognise are affecting our thoughts and behaviours. Addressing or receiving training around our unconscious biases is found to be an effective tool In addressing all areas of discrimination (Lane, 2021). The most significant reason that people experiencing mental health issues or are in crisis do not seek help or support is due to stigma (Smith-Frigerio, 2020), and for people from marginalised groups, this stigma could be perceived or experienced for multiple reasons, including having a mental health issue. Improving communication in mass and social media about mental health could improve the health outcomes of those from marginalised groups, in particular, who may be experiencing mental health concerns (Smith-Frigerio, 2020). Mental health professionals can increase and perpetuate the levels of stigma and discrimination experienced by those with mental health issues but it has been found that clinicians who are more experienced appear to stigmatise their clients less, likely because they have witnessed more recovery and have more experience in over-riding stigmatising attitudes (Henderson et al., 2022). More experienced clinicians have also worked with a lot of different people and are likely to have developed more significant levels of cultural competence just by having worked with people from various backgrounds. There has been a focus in healthcare on clinicians understanding stigma reduction, but there should be greater efforts to ensure clinicians are 'antistigma agents' (Henderson et al., 2022) and this means not only avoiding stigmatising attitudes within yourself but actively challenging and addressing stigma and discrimination when you witness it.

Activity

A term that has been mentioned several times is 'unconscious bias'. Take some time to think about each of the protected characteristic groups below and think of any beliefs, attitudes or stereotypes you may hold. This is a challenging exercise but it is important to be honest with yourself as simply saying 'I don't see colour' or 'I treat everyone the same' is avoiding the issue and ultimately not respecting that people do have differences in terms of culture and heritage that these terms dismiss.

- Age
- Disability
- Gender reassignment
- Marriage and civil partnership
- Pregnancy and maternity
- Race
- Religion or belief
- Sex
- Sexual orientation

As you have worked through each characteristic and group, you may have identified positive associations as well as negative stereotypes. Take some time to question both the positive and negative associations you made. Where do you think those thoughts have come from? Why do you think you hold that view? Do you think that is accurate or representative of the whole group? Have you had different perceptions of groups you identify with?

Again, this activity is challenging but that is the purpose! We need to first understand our own unconscious bias and examine it before we can move forward.

There are many situations where we could witness or experience discrimination, and what we do about that can be confusing or difficult to understand. As healthcare professionals, we should see ourselves as an ally to all marginalised groups and work to be antiracist and antidiscriminatory rather than simply not engaging in those behaviours ourselves. Consider the scenario's below and how you may approach them:

- One of your colleagues has just been called a racial slur by a client in your care.
- A client who is older has just been referred to as a 'little old dear' by one of your team.
- You have observed a staff member saying that they wouldn't keep any sandwiches for a client who is observing Ramadan as 'they should just eat with everyone else'.

- Your manager is repeatedly and deliberately misgendering a Trans client in front of staff and service users.
- A client who experiences chronic pain has cancelled their appointment as they can't come to the clinic, and your colleague has expressed their frustration that they've failed to attend another appointment and is thinking of discharging them from the service.

It can be confronting to witness these events but we must consider how it feels to experience them and the effects they can have on people. To be an ally, we must take action when we see discrimination in any form and so below are some suggestions of actions you could take in each scenario:

- Talk to your colleague. Tell them that you heard what was said and that you are sorry they were spoken to like that. Ask them how they are feeling and if there is anything you can do to support them. Offer to complete the incident form or talk to the client directly to explain that their conduct is inappropriate and unacceptable. Allow your colleague to express their feelings and lead the situation in terms of what happens next. They may want to escalate the situation or not; that is their decision and the most important thing is to let them know that they are supported.
- Talk to your colleague. Explain to them that that language is not appropriate and diminishes the client. They may have intended it in a positive way but that comment is belittling and patronising.
- Talk to your colleague. Explain that Ramadan is an important religious festival, and those who observe it, do not eat during daylight hours. Ultimately, withholding food in this way is not just discrimination, but it is also abusive. If they do not understand and correct their behaviour, escalate the situation immediately and ensure that food is provided for anyone who will be breaking a fast during the night.
- Talk to your colleague. Address how inappropriate it is to deliberately misgender anyone and explain how this is not treating them with respect and dignity. Personally, after addressing it directly, if they continued to misgender someone, I would correct them each time until they stopped. Again, it is not just discriminatory but incredibly traumatising for the client, so the conversation needs to be around respect, dignity and role-modelling to others. If they continue to behave in this manner or do not immediately correct their behaviour, then it should be escalated immediately.
- Talk to your colleague. The client experiences chronic pain; has your colleague considered the impact on their mobility or ability to attend a clinic physically? If they have repeatedly not attended, it may be because their physical health means they cannot attend. Ask your colleague if they have considered any adjustments to support their client, like doing a home visit instead or asking the client if particular times of day are better or worse for them. Support them to think about how they could approach the situation differently so that the client can receive and engage in their care.

As we can see, there is a common thread to all my suggestions above! Talking to people when you observe discrimination or poor attitudes in any form is crucial. It can take significant courage to speak up and challenge others but if we are to be an ally, that is what we must do.

Reflect on a time when someone has made you uncomfortable, someone approaching you to say 'I saw that, it wasn't ok, how are you feeling?' would have been a positive thing to experience wouldn't it? As mental health professionals, we should see ourselves as allies and antistigma agents. Taking time to consider our attitudes and biases is important but listening to others is more important. We do not have to be experts on all aspects that could form part of someone's identity but if we treat everyone with respect and dignity and listen to their experiences and needs, that is how we move forward.

References

Aharon, O.N., Aisenberg-Shafran, D. and Levi-Belz, Y. (2023) 'The effect of suicide severity and patient's age on mental health professionals' willingness to treat: The moderating effect of ageism', *Death Studies*, 86(1), pp. 1–11. doi:10.1080/07481187.2023.2255854.

Bailey, D. et al. (2022) 'Equal but different! improving care for older LGBT+ adults', *Age and Ageing*, 51(6). doi:10.1093/ageing/afac142.

Bernard, D.L. et al. (2020) 'Making the "C-ace" for a culturally-informed adverse childhood experiences framework to understand the pervasive mental health impact of racism on black youth', *Journal of Child & Adolescent Trauma*, 14(2), pp. 233–247. doi:10.1007/s40653-020-00319-9.

Bialer, P.A. and McIntosh, C.A. (2017) 'Discrimination and LGBT mental health', *Journal of Gay & Lesbian Mental Health*, 21(4), pp. 275–276. doi:10.1080/19359705.2017.1356138.

Brown, R.L. and Ciciurkaite, G. (2022) 'Disability, discrimination, and mental health during the COVID-19 pandemic: A stress process model', *Society and Mental Health*, 12(3), p. 215686932211153. doi:10.1177/21568693221115347.

Bryan, A. and Mayock, P. (2016) 'Supporting LGBT lives? complicating the suicide consensus in LGBT Mental Health Research', *Sexualities*, 20(1–2), pp. 65–85. doi:10.1177/1363460716648099.

Desai, M.U. et al. (2023) '"That was a state of depression by itself dealing with society": Atmospheric racism, mental health, and the black and african american faith community', *American Journal of Community Psychology*, 73(1–2), pp. 104–117. doi:10.1002/ajcp.12654.

Equality Act (2010) *Legislation.gov.uk*. Available at: https://www.legislation.gov.uk/ukpga/2010/15/section/4 (Accessed: 17 May 2024).

Henderson, C. et al. (2022) 'Training for mental health professionals in responding to experienced and anticipated mental health-related discrimination (Read-MH): Protocol for an international multisite feasibility study', *Pilot and Feasibility Studies*, 8(1). doi:10.1186/s40814-022-01208-8.

Hosang, G.M. and Bhui, K. (2018) 'Gender discrimination, victimisation and women's mental health', *The British Journal of Psychiatry*, 213(6), pp. 682–684. doi:10.1192/bjp.2018.244.

Kruse, S.D., Rakha, S. and Calderone, S. (2017) 'Developing cultural competency in higher education: An agenda for practice', *Teaching in Higher Education*, 23(6), pp. 733–750. doi:10.1080/13562517.2017.1414790.

Kucharska, J. (2017) 'Cumulative trauma, gender discrimination and mental health in women: Mediating role of self-esteem', *Journal of Mental Health*, 27(5), pp. 416–423. doi:10.1080/09638237.2017.1417548.

Kung, W.W. and Johansson, S. (2022) 'Ethical Mental Health Practice in diverse cultures and races', *Journal of Ethnic & Cultural Diversity in Social Work*, 31(3–5), pp. 248–262. doi:10.1080/15313204.2022.2070889.

Lane, C. (2021) 'Busting barriers to inclusivity: what some of them they are and how you can break them', *OfficePro* 81(7), pp. 10–12. Available at: https://research.ebsco.com/linkprocessor/plink?id=0174200c-a0bf-32af-b0cd-9f2314de333c (Accessed: 17 May 2024).

Mental Health Foundation (2022) *Men and women: Statistics* www.mentalhealth.org.uk. Available at: https://www.mentalhealth.org.uk/explore-mental-health/statistics/men-women-statistics#:~:text=Women%20between%20the%20ages%20of (Accessed: 16 May 2024).

Namkung, E.H. and Carr, D. (2020) 'The psychological consequences of disability over the life course: Assessing the mediating role of perceived interpersonal discrimination', *Journal of Health and Social Behavior*, 61(2), pp. 190–207. doi:10.1177/0022146520921371.

Office for National Statistics (2021) *Religion, England and Wales - Office for National Statistics*. www.ons.gov.uk. Available at: https://www.ons.gov.uk/peoplepopulationandcommunity/culturalidentity/religion/bulletins/religionenglandandwales/census2021 (Accessed: 16 May 2024).

Scheitle, C.P., Frost, J. and Ecklund, E.H. (2023) 'The association between religious discrimination and health: disaggregating by types of discrimination experiences, religious tradition, and forms of health', *Journal for the Scientific Study of Religion*, 62(4). doi:https://doi.org/10.1111/jssr.12871.

Seiler-Ramadas, R. et al. (2021) 'Strategies to challenge discrimination and foster inclusivity for LGBT+Q+ youth in workplaces: A qualitative exploratory study in six European countries', *European Journal of Public Health*, 31(Supplement_3). doi:10.1093/eurpub/ckab164.471.

Simela, C. et al. (2024) 'Intergenerational consequences of racism in the United Kingdom: A qualitative investigation into parents' exposure to racism and offspring mental health and well-being', *Child and Adolescent Mental Health*, 29(2), pp. 181–191. doi:10.1111/camh.12695.

Simon, K.M. (2023) 'Mitigating the negative mental health impact of racism on black adolescents – A preventive perspective', *JAMA Network Open*, 6(11). doi:10.1001/jamanetworkopen.2023.40577.

Smith-Frigerio, S. (2020) 'Grassroots Mental Health Groups' use of advocacy strategies in social media messaging', *Qualitative Health Research*, 30(14), pp. 2205–2216. doi:10.1177/1049732320951532.

Sutter, M. and Perrin, P.B. (2016) 'Discrimination, mental health, and suicidal ideation among LGBTQ people of color', *Journal of Counseling Psychology*, 63(1), pp. 98–105. doi:10.1037/cou0000126.

Vogt Yuan, A.S. (2007) 'Perceived age discrimination and mental health', *Social Forces*, 86(1), pp. 291–311. doi:10.1353/sof.2007.0113.

Whaibeh, E., Mahmoud, H. and Vogt, E.L. (2019) 'Reducing the treatment gap for LGBT mental health needs: The potential of telepsychiatry', *The Journal of Behavioral Health Services & Research*, 47(3), pp. 424–431. doi:10.1007/s11414-019-09677-1.

Williams, D.R. and Etkins, O.S. (2021) 'Racism and mental health', *World Psychiatry*, 20(2), pp. 194–195. doi:10.1002/wps.20845.

Williams, M.L. et al. (2022) 'The effect of the brexit vote on the variation in race and religious hate crimes in England, Wales, Scotland and Northern Ireland', *The British Journal of Criminology*, 63(4). doi:10.1093/bjc/azac071.

Wu, Z. and Schimmele, C.M. (2019) 'Perceived religious discrimination and mental health', *Ethnicity & Health*, 26(7), pp. 1–18. doi:10.1080/13557858.2019.1620176.

CHAPTER 9

Managing Therapeutic Relationships

Therapeutic relationships are crucial to any clinician's care and practice in mental health services (Brown and Parry, 2022), but understanding what they are, how to develop them, maintain them and end them positively and constructively can be complex and challenging. Engaging effectively with clients is core to the underpinning principles of all health and social care professions (Hartley et al., 2020). Engaging with clients is the beginning of a therapeutic relationship. Working together in a collaborative and consistent way is a crucial feature of a good therapeutic relationship (Brown and Parry, 2022). While it is generally accepted by all health and social care professionals that a good therapeutic relationship is important, developing and maintaining a therapeutic relationship can be a complex process (Tolosa-Merlos et al., 2022). One of the reasons that establishing and maintaining an excellent therapeutic relationship can be challenging is that each therapeutic relationship between a professional and client will be unique (Hartley et al., 2020). For this reason, we can consider broad principles, but how they are applied will depend on the clinician and the client that they are working with at that time. Another reason that therapeutic relationships can be challenging from a clinician's perspective is that many clients whom we will work within mental health services have experienced poor interpersonal relationships and trauma in their past, and therefore can find developing a positive therapeutic relationship challenging (Evans, 2022). This can be because they have not had positive, supportive or understanding relationships previously and can struggle to conceptualise how that feels and what that may look like. At the core of any therapeutic relationship is an interpersonal interaction between a client and a healthcare professional (Tolosa-Merlos et al., 2022) and when we consider that clients may have experienced very challenging interpersonal interactions, we can see how this becomes an important relationship to role model with clients and how it can have a significant impact on their future interpersonal interactions and relationships.

Thriving in Mental Health Nursing, First Edition. Laura Duncan.
© 2025 John Wiley & Sons Ltd. Published 2025 by John Wiley & Sons Ltd.

Research suggests that the quality of a therapeutic relationship (also known as a therapeutic alliance) is a more significant predictor of clinical outcomes than the therapeutic intervention (such as medication, therapy, etc.) itself (Romeu-Labayen et al., 2020). The evidence for positive therapeutic relationships improving outcomes consistently has been evidenced in all types of services and interventions (Brown and Parry, 2022) and a poor or negative therapeutic relationship can lead to treatment being ended or disengagement from services (Evans, 2022). Therefore, we should view therapeutic relationships as a form of treatment within themselves (Evans, 2022) as a good therapeutic relationship has been found to increase engagement as well as improve outcomes (Brown and Parry, 2022) for the client.

There are a number of potential barriers to creating a positive therapeutic relationship such as time limitations, staffing shortages and the volume of tasks that may need to be completed but when the therapeutic relationship is lacking, clients can feel that the professionals are uninvolved or uncaring (Tolosa-Merlos et al., 2022). Professionals can also find it very challenging to manage multiple therapeutic relationships simultaneously, particularly when they are emotionally difficult or complex and this can lead to feeling burned out as a clinician (Hartley et al., 2020). This highlights the importance of considering how developing and maintaining a therapeutic relationship may impact a professional as an individual and utilise supervision and case discussions to ensure that the professional's well-being is being maintained, particularly when working with lots of clients or clients that may be very complex in terms of their needs.

So, we have established that developing and maintaining a therapeutic relationship is important and challenging, but what does a 'good' therapeutic relationship look like? As mentioned above, each therapeutic relationship will be unique, and this is important to recognise as all clients' value being known and understood as individual human being (Hartley et al., 2020). A key feature of good therapeutic relationships is developing trust and understanding between a client and professional (Brown and Parry, 2022). Core traits of good therapeutic relationships include compassion, acceptance, honesty, warmth and hope (Romeu-Labayen et al., 2020). Normalising experiences, particularly of psychosis but all mental health issues can help develop a supportive therapeutic relationship (Brown and Parry, 2022) and this can also be part of psychoeducation where we explain to clients who may be experiencing particular symptoms or a specific diagnosis what that means, that other people have also experienced this and that they can recover and feel better. This not only normalises their (often frightening and distressing) symptoms but also communicates your experience and knowledge as a professional, which helps to develop trust, inspires hope and follows the recovery model. Feeling listened to is another essential component of building trust within a therapeutic relationship. Validating someone's experiences as their thoughts and feelings can be very powerful in developing a therapeutic relationship. Research has also found that creating a 'safe space to talk' is crucial in developing a therapeutic relationship, and two other factors that are core to positive outcomes are developing a 'sense of trust' and taking a 'nonjudgmental approach' (Brown and Parry, 2022).

Another critical consideration in a positive therapeutic relationship is maintaining appropriate boundaries; professionals must always be mindful of this within a therapeutic relationship

(Evans, 2022). Core to this is understanding that a therapeutic relationship is not the same as a 'friend' relationship, as the focus is not on mutual support or fun but on the client and their needs. This can be a difficult concept to understand, particularly for those developing their professional identities early in their career. Ultimately, as a professional, this relationship is not about you or your needs and the client should always be at the centre of it. There are some clinical environments, such as forensic mental health services, where the need to maintain physical safety can overshadow the development of a therapeutic relationship and restrictive practices such as physical restraint of service users can actively damage the development or continuation of a therapeutic relationship (Moyles, Hunter and Grealish, 2023). We must also acknowledge an inherent power imbalance within a therapeutic relationship (Moyles, Hunter and Grealish, 2023) and as the professional, you are the one in a position of authority. However, this can be addressed positively by naming this power imbalance and acknowledging it. This imbalance can feel most acute within inpatient services, mainly when the client is detained under the Mental Health Act (1983) and their freedoms are substantially limited. Acknowledging that this is the situation but focussing on how to move forward collaboratively can be very powerful in establishing a strong therapeutic relationship.

Activities

When we think about a therapeutic relationship, it has a natural progression to it. This can be separated into the 'development', 'maintenance' and 'ending' stages and within this activity, we will consider what is important within each stage to consider.

Developing a Therapeutic Relationship

Within the initial stages of developing a therapeutic relationship first we must consider the clinical environment we are working within as this will have a significant impact on how we commence a therapeutic relationship and what the goals for that client will be. In some clinical environments, the therapeutic relationship will last briefly, whereas in others, it will span months or even years. Knowing what is likely in terms of duration is important at the outset of a therapeutic relationship as it will help us to manage expectations effectively, which in itself builds trust and understanding. For professionals working in crisis or assessment-based environments, such as psychiatric liaison, primary care or liaison and diversion services, it can be difficult to conceptualise such a short working period with an individual to constitute a therapeutic relationship, however, it will still follow the same structure as a more prolonged therapeutic relationship. It will share the same features, so for all intents and purposes, it is a therapeutic relationship even if it only lasts for 20 minutes!

At the very beginning of any therapeutic relationship comes our introductions. We need to ensure we are introducing ourselves effectively, and this includes:

- Giving our name and how we would like to be addressed and asking the client how they would like to be addressed. It is the basis of all future interactions and should not be underestimated in terms of its importance. Consider how you would feel if you would prefer to be addressed as 'Mr/Mrs/Ms/Mx X', and someone presumed they could call you by your first name; you would find it rude and probably not immediately warm to that person. While most people are fine with being addressed by their first name, many are not and we cannot presume this. Many people also prefer a specific version of their name, so asking explicitly 'How would you like me to address you?' allows the client to share their preferred name or pronouns and immediately sets the relationship off on a respectful tone.

- Explaining our role, the service and its parameters. Depending upon the clinical environment, we need to ensure the client understands who we are, why we are there, how the service works and what the boundaries of that service are. It is easy to forget when you are a professional that the set-up of services can be very confusing for clients, particularly when they have never accessed that service previously. If we are working in an assessment-based service, we can explain that our role is to try and understand what is happening for them and how we can help. We will then refer them to appropriate services that can support them on a longer term basis. If we work in inpatient services, many clients will not understand the nature of shift work. A basic explanation of how there will be different staff each day/night but that there will always be someone they can approach if they need anything can be very reassuring. It also establishes that you will not be there 24/7 and clarifies that boundary from the outset to prevent misunderstandings or the client feeling abandoned or upset at you leaving at the end of your shift. If working in the community, we may be working with that client on a much longer term basis, so explaining the parameters of that is important. We should define the frequency of meetings that we anticipate, other members of the team and their roles in supporting them and what happens out of hours, in the event of a crisis or if you are on leave/leave the service.

- When establishing our therapeutic relationship in this manner, we must also consider whether we are having these conversations in a 'safe space'. Think about privacy, can others hear what is being said? Are you likely to be interrupted? Is the space comfortable physically? We need to ensure that we can both 'hear' and 'be heard', so try to use an environment that is quiet and relaxing. This can be challenging in certain environments but it is essential to make these considerations and try to implement them to the best of our abilities.

- Give time and space. In our initial interaction with a client, we need to establish their experiences and needs. Many individuals accessing mental health services in any context will have experienced a tough time in the run-up to that first meeting. We need to consider that we may be the first person that they have disclosed what is happening; they may be frightened of what will happen if they tell you how they have been feeling, or they may struggle to verbalise their thoughts and feelings. That is why giving time to allow them to disclose what they are comfortable with at their own pace is important.

- Validate their feelings. When you have worked with many clients with similar concerns, it can be easy to forget how difficult it can be to feel the way the client is feeling. There are simple phrases that can demonstrate you understand and validate their thoughts and feelings, such as 'that must have been really hard for you', 'that sounds really tough' or 'I'm sorry that you have been feeling like this'. Of course, this should be genuine as a response, so phrasing this in a natural way to you as an individual is important.

- Use active listening skills. Good communication skills are important in all components of clinical practice, but during the development of a therapeutic relationship, it is especially important to utilise active listening skills to ensure the client feels heard and understood effectively. These skills can include considering our body language, ensuring it is 'open' (i.e. not crossing arms or legs, etc.), that we are sat at an appropriate distance (not too close to feel as though we are intruding on their personal space but not so far that it feels there is a significant distance between us and the client) and making appropriate eye contact (not staring but not looking down or away). Active listening also gives the client time and space to talk, not rushing or interrupting and allowing silence. Silence can be very uncomfortable, but it is important not to fill silence ourselves as it may impede the client from sharing something they may have needed time to think about or express. Summarising and clarifying points are also an important facet of active listening to ensure you accurately understand what the individual has shared. This can sometimes feel uncomfortable, particularly when we are new to using these skills but using phrases such as 'From what you've said, I understood that you are feeling "X" about "X," is that correct?' allows the client to address any misunderstandings immediately and shows that you have been listening to what they have said to you, which is not to be underestimated in terms of its significance.

- At the end of our initial meeting, it is important to establish a plan moving forward. This could be when you will next meet with them, what the next step will be or what happens next such as 'I'll show you to your bedroom and then around the ward'. This is a time to establish a plan of action so the client knows what to expect, such as a referral to another service or team member, discharge, or next steps on the ward, such as meal times, etc. When ending the initial interaction, express that you are glad they spoke to you so openly, thank them for meeting with you, or reassure them that you and the team are there to support them and help them feel better ensure that you end the initial interaction on a positive note and conveys your respect to them as an individual.

Maintaining a Therapeutic Relationship

- Now we have established a therapeutic relationship effectively, we need to ensure we positively maintain this. The key to this is being honest and transparent. We need to ensure that we have explained the boundaries of our role effectively so that the client is aware of when and how we will be available and when we will not. For example, if you are working with a client in the community and your working pattern is Monday–Friday, 9–5, it would be inappropriate to advise a client that you are available 24/7 if they need you. Being honest about 'I work from 9 a.m.–5 p.m., I may be with other clients or in meetings so I can't promise you I will always be able to answer the phone immediately, but I will call you back as soon as I am able to. If you need help or support outside of my working hours, please contact the crisis team via "X" phone number' not only establishes an appropriate and professional boundary but communicates your role effectively so that the client understands and will not later be disappointed or upset that you didn't answer their call immediately or at 3 p.m. on a Saturday. By being honest and transparent in this manner, we build trust and by following up on our agreements regarding returning calls, etc., we develop and maintain that sense of confidence and respect.
- Be goal focussed. Once you have established what is important to the client regarding their recovery and how they would like their future to look, review this with them regularly to ensure that you remain aligned with them regarding the ultimate goal.
- Remain positive and hopeful. Recovery is not linear and clients will experience relapses, new symptoms or other challenges; so, working with them through this is important and being the person who reassures them that they will move past this is powerful.

- Be honest. If you think there needs to be a change of plan regarding their treatment, be truthful about this. If you think they need another service, discuss this openly with them and why, in your professional opinion, this needs to happen and how you anticipate it will benefit them.
- Communicate effectively. If you need to cancel an appointment, an emergency has happened and you won't make your visit, you are off sick etc, communicate this as early as possible and understand that this can be upsetting to the client. They may have been waiting to see you because they are worried about something or have rearranged other things to be present for your meeting and so cancelling or changing plans can be very frustrating. If you acknowledge this and apologise for any inconvenience or upset, this will go a long way in maintaining a positive and constructive therapeutic relationship.

Ending a Therapeutic Relationship

- Therapeutic relationships will naturally end, either because the client no longer needs our service and can be discharged or their needs change and a different service is more appropriate. We may also come to the end of our role in terms of why we are working with that individual, so acknowledging that all therapeutic relationships will come to an end is important.
- When discharging a client, it is important to do this in a structured manner. If we have worked with someone for a long time, it can be very daunting for a client not to be engaged with a service any longer, even if it is because they are doing really well and in a much more positive place. We should acknowledge that discharge is the ultimate goal for them, and as soon as we think we are approaching that, we should discuss that with the client and recognize their feelings about it.
- When discharging or transitioning to another service, it is important to try and make that as smooth as possible. Using the example of a client working with child and adolescent services and moving to adult services, we can see how difficult that transition could be for the client. Good planning of this transition is crucial, and introducing them to the team they will be working with in the future and effectively 'co-working' for a few months is an excellent idea that will facilitate a smooth transition and support the new team in developing a positive therapeutic relationship but also will ensure the client feels well supported.
- When ending a therapeutic relationship, ensure the client knows what to do if they feel they need additional support again and that they are aware of any crisis or safety plans they may need.
- Say goodbye and acknowledge that it can be difficult or emotional to end a therapeutic relationship but that it is ultimately a positive thing due to them being in a better place or needing a different type of support that you and your service can't offer. Hence, it is the best thing to ensure they have appropriate support for their needs.

Acknowledging when we have done an excellent job at building, maintaining and ending a therapeutic relationship can be one of the most rewarding parts of a professional's role. Knowing that the client had a more positive experience and outcome because we had an excellent therapeutic relationship is incredibly powerful. Using our reflection skills to understand when this has gone well and how we can do it better is an integral part of our clinical practice throughout our careers.

References

Brown, K. and Parry, S. (2022) 'How do people with first episode psychosis experience therapeutic relationships with mental health practitioners? A narrative review', *Psychosis*, pp. 1–12. doi:10.1080/17522439.2022.2160487.

Department of Health (1983) *The Mental Health Act* available at https://www.legislation.gov.uk/ukpga/1983/20 (Accessed: 29 April 2024).

Evans, N. (2022) 'Why the nurse-patient relationship is key in mental healthcare', *Mental Health Practice*, 25(6), pp. 12–13. doi:10.7748/mhp.25.6.12.s6.

Hartley, S. et al. (2020) 'Effective nurse–patient relationships in mental health care: A systematic review of interventions to improve the therapeutic alliance', *International Journal of Nursing Studies*, 102, p. 103490. doi:10.1016/j.ijnurstu.2019.103490.

Moyles, J., Hunter, A. and Grealish, A. (2023) 'Forensic mental health nurses' experiences of rebuilding the therapeutic relationship after an episode of physical restraint in forensic services in Ireland: A qualitative study', *International Journal of Mental Health Nursing*. doi:10.1111/inm.13176.

Romeu-Labayen, M. et al. (2020) 'Borderline personality disorder in a community setting: Service users' experiences of the therapeutic relationship with mental health nurses', *International Journal of Mental Health Nursing*, 29(5), pp. 868–877. doi:10.1111/inm.12720.

Tolosa-Merlos, D. et al. (2022) 'The therapeutic relationship at the heart of nursing care: A participatory action research in acute mental health units', *Journal of Clinical Nursing*, 32(15–16), pp. 5135–5146. doi:10.1111/jocn.16606.

CHAPTER 10

Managing Complexity

Complexity when it comes to mental health care is, unsurprisingly, a complex issue! When we refer to complexity in mental health, we usually mean an individual with additional needs or diagnoses, but complexity can also exist where there are environmental or behavioural issues that can be difficult to manage. In the literature, complexity in mental health may refer to additional physical health issues, intellectual and/or developmental disorders (IDDs) or substance misuse issues. Complexity can also be due to a client's age, such as children and adolescents and older adults, as these client groups can have specific and multifaceted needs. The reason that we need to consider the complexity and additional needs is that all aspects of someone's life need to be considered when trying to improve their mental health and wellbeing (Agerton and Iasiello, 2019). Comorbidity can be seen as one reason for 'complexity', but this is not the only reason, and comorbidities or additional conditions don't always impact case complexity (Gallant and Good, 2023).

A core issue with clients with complex needs is that when an individual has a higher number of additional needs, there is an increased risk of misdiagnosis or treatment interactions, which also means that a more complex care plan is necessary (Dunn et al., 2020) and this can mean a care plan that needs to work across multiple services. Research also suggests that there has been a marked increase in clients being admitted to mental health units with co-occurring mental health issues and substance misuse issues (Dugmore and Bauweraerts, 2021). We also see an increased rate of hospitalisation for individuals with both IDDs and mental health issues (Lineberry et al., 2023). Physical health issues are also more prevalent for clients with mental health issues, but depression is the second most prevalent comorbidity for those living with chronic obstructive pulmonary Disease (COPD) (Wang et al., 2021), which demonstrates that comorbidities can go both ways, with physical health issues leading to mental health/wellbeing issues and vice versa. Many people use smoking as a way to manage difficult emotions (Wang et al., 2021) and it is widely understood and accepted that the leading cause of the development of COPD is smoking. These considerations highlight the need for truly holistic and person-centred care that

Thriving in Mental Health Nursing, First Edition. Laura Duncan.
© 2025 John Wiley & Sons Ltd. Published 2025 by John Wiley & Sons Ltd.

considers the whole person and all of their needs equally rather than our clinical specialism – which means that the care we deliver can become siloed and fragmented.

Mental health issues in children and adolescents can have a significant impact on their social, academic and community engagement (Gallant and Good, 2023) which can have a lasting effect on their health and social needs in adulthood. Childhood abuse and adverse childhood experiences (ACEs) have been linked to an increased risk of depression and alcohol consumption during adolescence which is strongly correlated to an increased risk of substance misuse and mental health issues in adulthood (Skinner et al., 2016). There can be significant consequences for children and young people if their mental health needs are unmet, including social exclusion and poor academic attainment (Gallant and Good, 2023). Poor academic attainment can have a long-lasting impact on an individual including their employment and educational options in adulthood. We also see that individuals with autistic spectrum disorder (ASD) are believed to experience a greater number of ACEs which could have a negative impact on future physical and mental health outcomes later in life (Kerns et al., 2017). IDDs were previously believed to mean that individuals with IDDs could not also have mental health issues, but research has now evidenced that this is not the case, and individuals with IDD actually have higher prevalence rates of mental health issues than the general population (Lineberry et al., 2023). It is believed that individuals with ASD are more likely to experience co-occurring mental health issues, which can cause greater challenges and difficulties for this client group, but this could be linked to being more likely to have experienced ACEs (Kerns et al., 2017). One reason that mental health issues and complexities/comorbidities are poorly understood for those with IDD is communication variances within this population. Individuals who communicate without speech are more likely to not have any mental health diagnosis, and this may be due to the complexity of understanding someone's emotional state without explicit verbal communication (Lineberry et al., 2023) rather than the actual absence of a mental health condition. Research also suggests that vision and hearing loss are more common for those with IDD or ASD (Dunn et al., 2020) which can significantly add to communication complexity. Communication challenges are not exclusive to those with IDD or ASD, however, and it is believed that one key aspect that can add to complexity for clients with Dementia is impaired communication as well as reduced insight and capacity (Jones et al., 2022).

For those with multiple conditions or additional complexities, due to the need for multiple different services to support them, the coordination of their care can become very complex and lead to poorer outcomes or standards of care (Dunn et al., 2020). We find that inter-agency working still faces challenges with clients with complex needs feeling that they are blocked from accessing specialist services due to their multiple or complex needs (Allen et al., 2024). Care for young people can feel very fragmented (Gallant and Good, 2023) but this can also be true for anyone with multiple services needing to be involved in their care. Historically, there has been poor communication and inter-agency working between mental health and substance misuse services (Dugmore and Bauweraerts, 2021) and despite the prevalence of clients that need support from both services, there appears to have been little improvement in this area. We also see that there is limited mental health training for physical health clinicians (Wang et al., 2021) to support them in understanding how to identify clients who may have mental health or wellbeing issues and how/who to refer to appropriately. Diagnostic overshadowing is also a significant concern for clients with ASD as many additional conditions or pain responses are not explored or considered appropriately due to a client having ASD (Woods, Williams and Watts, 2023) but diagnostic overshadowing is also a serious issue for all those with mental health issues or IDD, more generally. Mental health services can be difficult to access, and other services tend to feel there is a lack of collaborative working, but this is likely due to mental health services being unable to keep up with demand due to increased levels of need without increased staffing or service provision (Allen et al., 2024). This does appear to be an issue across the health and social care sector however. As we can see, there needs to be greater inter-professional collaboration to support clients with comorbidities (Wang et al., 2021) and the variety of comorbidities and complexities means that 'inter-professional' ultimately means being able to work with all health and social care professionals across the sector. One key way to address this is through training and education, as inter-professional staff training has been shown to increase communication and joint working (Dugmore and Bauweraerts, 2021), and ideally, this should occur as early in the career of professionals as possible.

Another key factor in addressing and mitigating comorbidities and complexities is early intervention and considering family and carers within service provision. For families where there are complex issues present such as abuse, mental health or substance misuse issues, early intervention is critical as this can prevent issues from becoming more entrenched over time (Allen et al., 2024). We also see that in regards to Dementia specifically, in later stages up to 90% of individuals are believed to experience behaviour changes such as agitation, restlessness or continence issues which can be seen to add to the complexity of their care but a significant reason for inpatient admissions for this client group is carer exhaustion or a lack of or deterioration of the support system they may have at home (Jones et al., 2022). From this, we can see that it is not only important to work holistically with the individual in terms of their needs but to also to consider the whole family and support network of the client.

Activity

Consider your specialist area and where your particular strengths are for clients as an individual and service

- How would you support a client who you believed had additional needs in relation to:
  - Their physical health.
  - Having an IDD.
  - Substance/alcohol misuse issues.
  - ASD.
  - Other neurodivergent conditions such as attention deficit hyperactivity disorder, attention deficit disorder, dyslexia or dyscalculia

- Having a complex family unit or safeguarding needs.
    - Having communication difficulties such as being unable to communicate verbally.
- Do you have clear referral pathways and inter-agency working for clients with the above needs?
- How would you provide holistic care for someone whose behaviour you found to be very challenging?
- How would you support clinicians from other specialisms who felt an individual would benefit from your care?

We see clearly throughout the literature that individuals can be very complex, and there are multiple issues that can come from that, including poorer outcomes, diagnostic overshadowing and being unable to access services that are required. We also see that from a clinician's perspective, it can be incredibly challenging to identify clinical needs outside of your own area of specialism but that inter-agency and inter-professional communication can be a significant challenge. There is a need for greater integration of services in primary, secondary and tertiary health and social care services and this will hopefully be addressed more effectively in the coming years. As individual clinicians, we must be working holistically with the client and their support network to ensure that all additional needs and requirements are identified with appropriate support given. I have heard too frequently 'I'm a mental health nurse, I don't do physical health' (and the same with other professions in relation to mental health!) which is the antithesis of the attitude we should hold. We are all responsible for ensuring a client has good outcomes not just in terms of their mental health but also their holistic health and social needs so that individuals can thrive and achieve true wellbeing.

Vignette

To highlight the need to consider someone's physical health needs as well as their mental health needs, the following vignette took place when I was a support worker working on a psychiatric intensive care unit (PICU).

Benny was a male in his mid-30s who had a long-standing diagnosis of schizophrenia and had experienced multiple inpatient admissions, many requiring a transfer to PICU to support his needs effectively. During this particular admission, Benny had been on the ward for several weeks at this time. Benny was a larger gentleman with a high body mass index (BMI) and large waist circumference, increasing his risk of physical health issues due to obesity. Benny also smoked cigarettes and would eat and drink excessively. Benny routinely refused physical health observations which were always offered on admission to PICU and then weekly throughout someone's admission. As a support worker, at that time, I had had very limited physical health training and had been taught to undertake physical health observations on the ward by the nursing team. I attended a physical health training session that was provided by the trust I worked for at the time, and there was a strong focus on diabetes, due to the prevalence of diabetes for clients with mental health issues and the impact of certain antipsychotic medication (such as olanzapine and clozapine) on blood glucose levels.

Whilst the training was ongoing and the Nurses leading the training were discussing the key symptoms of diabetes, I remember thinking, 'Benny has all of those symptoms!' He was frequently requesting additional drinks because he felt thirsty all the time, he was urinating throughout the night, and he also reported being hungry and tired almost every time you spoke to him. I remember feeling almost panicked. It seemed to be clear that he had all of the warning signs of diabetes. I was on shift the next day and approached the nurse-in-charge, feeding back what I had learned and my concerns about Benny. They agreed that it seemed very likely Benny had diabetes but that he had always refused to have any blood taken, including for blood glucose monitoring. We discussed the situation, and we agreed that I would try to work with Benny throughout the day to check his blood glucose levels. We had a very good therapeutic relationship and so I was confident that I could work effectively with him in this situation.

I spoke at length with Benny and explained clearly why I was concerned and that if he did have diabetes, there were lots of treatment options available that would help him to feel better. I explained that I thought his feelings of tiredness, thirst and hunger could all be linked to Diabetes but that we needed to check his blood sugars with a small finger prick. Benny had fixed delusions about clinicians being vampires and that was why they were always asking for blood samples; so, I reassured him that it was literally a drop of blood and that he would see me dispose of the testing strip that had the blood immediately after. He didn't believe me that it was only a drop of blood and wasn't going to involve a cut to his finger or anything of that nature so we agreed that I would show him exactly the process and procedure first by doing it on myself. He agreed that if he saw me do it and it was only a drop of blood, he would agree to the procedure. I explained to him the normal ranges for blood glucose before we started as I was concerned his paranoid ideation around blood may mean that he thought I had changed the parameters based on his result. I told him that the meter should read between 4 and 7 and that anything outside of that would mean we needed to talk to the doctor. He understood and agreed to the plan, as long as I went first!

I performed the test on myself, and unexpectedly, my blood sugar reading was 2.7 mmols! When he saw the result, Benny said 'So that means you need to see a doctor, right?', I agreed that I did and that I would arrange that for myself the following day when I was not working! He then agreed to his sample, and it was 11.4 mmols. He understood immediately that it was higher than it should be and that he needed to speak to the doctor about the next steps.

Obviously, my result being out of range was unintended (I had no idea I had low blood sugar until that moment!), but agreeing with him that I needed to see a doctor about my result, I think I made him feel better about his result having the same outcome. In this scenario, I think I communicated with Benny effectively so that he understood how concerned I was for his health and that I was trying to help him feel better. He did go on to be formally diagnosed with Type 2 Diabetes, and for the rest of the time I knew him, it was managed well with oral medication, and he did not require Insulin at that time.

In this vignette, it is clear how additional training led to an increased understanding for me as the clinician and how this then led to Benny receiving care that addressed his physical health needs. I communicated with him clearly and was transparent about every step of the process and what it meant so that he felt he could trust me. He did actually ask me the next time I was on shift if I had gone to a doctor, which I confirmed that I did, and the situation ultimately led to a strengthening of our therapeutic relationship.

References

Allen, K. et al. (2024) 'Experiences of current UK service provision for co-occurring parental domestic violence and abuse, mental ill-health, and substance misuse: A reflexive thematic analysis,' *Children and Youth Services Review*, 158, p. 107449. doi: 10.1016/j.childyouth.2024.107449.

Agteren, J. and Iasiello, M. (2019) 'Advancing our understanding of mental wellbeing and mental health: The call to embrace complexity over simplification', *Australian Psychologist*, 55(4). doi:10.1111/ap.12440.

Dugmore, L. and Bauweraerts, S. (2021) 'When policy fails try something different integrated practice improve outcomes for dual diagnosis co-occurring service users accessing mental health services,' *Drugs and Alcohol Today*, 21(2), pp. 157–170. doi:10.1108/dat-06-2020-0036.

Dunn, K., Rydzewska, E., Fleming, M. and Cooper, S.-A. (2020) 'Prevalence of mental health conditions, sensory impairments and physical disability in people with co-occurring intellectual disabilities and autism compared with other people: A cross-sectional total population study in Scotland', *BMJ Open*, 10(4), p. e035280. doi:10.1136/bmjopen-2019-035280.

Gallant, C. and Good, D. (2023) 'Mental health complexity among children and youth: Current conceptualizations and future directions', *Canadian Journal of Community Mental Health*, pp. 1–12. doi:10.7870/cjcmh-2023-018.

Jones, L., Cullum, N., Watson, R. and Keady, J. (2022) 'Introducing the "3 Fs model of complexity" for people with dementia accessing a NHS mental health in-patient dementia assessment ward: An interpretive description study', *Dementia*, p. 147130122211363. doi:10.1177/14713012221136313.

Kerns, C.M., Newschaffer, C.J., Berkowitz, S. and Lee, B.K. (2017) 'Brief report: Examining the association of autism and adverse childhood experiences in the national survey of children's health: The important role of income and co-occurring mental health conditions', *Journal of Autism and Developmental Disorders*, 47(7), pp. 2275–2281. doi:10.1007/s10803-017-3111-7.

Lineberry, S., Bogenschutz, M., Broda, M., Dinora, P., Prohn, S. and West, A. (2023) 'Co-occurring mental illness and behavioral support needs in adults with intellectual and developmental disabilities,' *Community Mental Health Journal* doi:10.1007/s10597-023-01091-4.

Skinner, M.L., Hong, S., Herrenkohl, T.I., Brown, E.C., Lee, J.O. and Jung, H. (2016) 'Longitudinal effects of early childhood maltreatment on co-occurring substance misuse and mental health problems in adulthood: The role of adolescent alcohol use and depression', *Journal of Studies on Alcohol and Drugs*, 77(3), pp. 464–472. doi:10.15288/jsad.2016.77.464.

Wang, J., Willis, K., Barson, E. and Smallwood, N. (2021) 'The complexity of mental health care for people with COPD: A qualitative study of clinicians' perspectives', *Primary Care Respiratory Medicine*, 31(1). doi:10.1038/s41533-021-00252-w.

Woods, R., Williams, K. and Watts, C. (2023) '"Profound autism": The dire consequences of diagnostic overshadowing,' *Autism Research: Official Journal of the International Society for Autism Research*, 16(9), pp. 1656–1657. doi: 10.1002/aur.2985.

CHAPTER 11

Conflict

Unfortunately, aggressive events and conflict are very common in mental health services, and this can cause significant emotional or physical harm (Price et al., 2018) to both staff and service users. Due to this, we can see the use of restrictive practices such as the use of seclusion, physical restraint or rapid tranquilisation and there is a significant need to find a way to avoid such restrictive practices due to the negative impact on both service users and staff (Pérez-Toribio et al., 2021). One impact of aggressive behaviour is a diminished therapeutic relationship (Brenig, Gade and Voellm, 2023) which has a negative impact on both clients and staff. Restrictive practices such as restraint and seclusion are both linked to significant harm, including injury, post-traumatic stress disorder and even death (Price et al., 2018). Restrictive measures are intended to be used when other preventative strategies, such as de-escalation, have not been effective, and there is an identified risk of harm if no further action is taken (Brenig, Gade and Voellm, 2023). However, the response to violence or aggression must be proportional (Hallett and Dickens, 2015) and so if there is no identified risk of physical harm, then physical intervention should be minimised. There is a consensus that internationally, restrictive practices are used too frequently and are not saved for 'last resort' as they should be in principle (Gildberg et al., 2021), with some clinicians appearing to believe that medications such as PRN (Pro Re Nata or 'as required') should be used as a de-escalation tool (Hallett and Dickens, 2015). All medication, however, comes with risk, particularly benzodiazepines, such as lorazepam, diazepam or clonazepam, which are frequently used as PRN in these scenarios, but we must remember they can cause significant issues, including addiction. Ultimately, the rate and level of restrictive practices being used indicate that de-escalation and effective conflict management skills are not being used as routinely or effectively as they could be (Price et al., 2018). The Service User experience of restrictive interventions is that they are frightening, confusing, painful and even dehumanising (Brenig, Gade and Voellm, 2023), which highlights the importance of minimising these practices as far as possible.

The ultimate way to prevent the escalation of conflict to a violent or aggressive situation is effective de-escalation of the situation. Positive therapeutic relationships are vital in preventing conflict in the first place (Gildberg et al., 2021) but having a positive therapeutic relationship can

Thriving in Mental Health Nursing, First Edition. Laura Duncan.
© 2025 John Wiley & Sons Ltd. Published 2025 by John Wiley & Sons Ltd.

help to manage and address the conflict quickly and efficiently if conflict or aggression does occur. De-escalation techniques are both verbal and non-verbal techniques that are intended to reduce aggression without using restrictive practices (Price et al., 2018). It is vital for successful de-escalation that the de-escalator controls their own emotions effectively and expresses respect and empathy for the client they are attempting to de-escalate (Brenig, Gade and Voellm, 2023). De-escalation should be non-confrontational (Hallett and Dickens, 2015) and there are core principles of de-escalation that include removing objects that could be used as weapons, maintaining exit routes, removing others that don't need to be present (including excessive numbers of staff as well as other service users) and attempting to resolve the issue that led to the agitation or aggression in the first place (Price et al., 2018). It is important to remember that staff and service user perceptions of what led to conflict or aggression can be very different, and ultimately staff and service user interactions are core factors in staff/service user conflict (Gildberg et al., 2021). Staff having poor or weak interpersonal skills is seen to be a key trigger of aggression from service users (Hallett and Dickens, 2015). This is why from a clinician's perspective, demonstrating respect and empathy are key to any de-escalation approach (Price et al., 2018). It is noted that some tactics that can be helpful include problem-solving, distraction, the removal of triggers or moving the client to a different area (Hallett and Dickens, 2015), which highlights the importance of using quiet or 'low stimuli' areas at the earliest opportunity when conflict arises. Another key approach that can assist in effective conflict management or de-escalation is staff having a dialogue with clients about their 'early warning signs' and how they would like to be approached as this has been shown to reduce the severity of aggression and the likelihood for restrictive practices to be used (Gildberg et al., 2021). Effective de-escalation has been found to improve the situation in 80% of incidents (Price et al., 2018) which highlights the importance of considering our own de-escalation skills and awareness of how we manage conflict as clinicians. It has been shown that nurses' tolerance levels for conflict appear to be a significant factor in how conflict is managed, with those having higher levels of tolerance approaching situations in a calmer and more informal manner (Gildberg et al., 2021). We also need to consider that good de-escalation skills require a sound understanding of the link between trauma and aggression (Brenig, Gade and Voellm, 2023), as those who have experienced significant trauma may struggle with managing their own feelings and emotions but also how they express them in a productive or appropriate manner.

Activity

Consider your own approaches to managing conflict:
- Think of an occasion when you have perceived someone to be becoming aggressive or hostile towards you:
  - What was your immediate thought? Did you want to leave the situation? If you did leave, do you think that helped to de-escalate the situation? If you didn't, what was your next step?

- What do you think led to the individual becoming aggressive or hostile? Was there anything that could have been identified earlier to prevent the situation from becoming more difficult?
- Do you think you were able to remain as calm as you would have liked?
- Do you think you demonstrated respect and empathy?
- What verbal and non-verbal skills do you think you used?
- How was the situation resolved?
- Did you have a debrief with the team and the individual about the situation?
- Did you learn anything that you could take forward with that client or, more generally, in similar situations in the future?

We have to remember as clinicians that we are still human beings who will have an emotional response to another person being hostile or violent towards us, themselves or others and learning to identify our own emotions and how they impact us and our behaviour is crucial in developing our professional skills.

The National Institute of Clinical Health and Excellence (NICE) has published guidelines regarding managing violent and aggressive behaviour in mental health environments (2015) that makes some important considerations.

NICE (2015) Guidelines recognise that initially we must anticipate and reduce the risk of violence and aggression and key points within that are as follows:

- Using a person-centred approach and involving individuals in decisions about their care, including risk management plans.
- Developing skills to recognise why someone may become aggressive or violent, including environmental factors such as physical restrictions of being admitted to an inpatient unit (for example).
- Having good de-escalation skills.
- Good staff emotional regulation, management and effective leadership.
- Recognising dynamics between clients.
- Consider personal dynamics outside of the clinical environment such as difficult family situations.
- PRN should not be used routinely or automatically and needs to be prescribed and administered with a clear rationale.
- Staff should be trained to recognise the early signs of agitation or conflict and be able to use distraction or calming strategies to avoid escalation or provocation.
- Incidents of violence and aggression should be reviewed carefully to establish if there are any lessons that can be learned from a team level but also an organisational level.
- De-escalation should be led by one staff member who continually assesses for safety, negotiates and uses communication skills to address the anxiety or frustration in an appropriate environment.

These key principles within NICE (2015) guidelines are helpful in understanding the key areas to focus on in order to avoid conflict in the first place. If we are able to establish positive therapeutic relationships with clients then that will immediately improve levels of conflict and escalation of situations. If we can discuss openly with individuals about things that may cause frustration or irritation to them and then plan for how to work together to manage that, again conflict is reduced. If we as staff can manage our own emotions and remain calm even when there is conflict, this will again help us to move forward and reduce the risk of escalation.

Ultimately, the earlier that irritation, frustration or anger can be identified, the easier it is to de-escalate effectively.

Case Study

Anita is a 28-year-old female who has been admitted to the unit following several incidents in the community where she has been behaving erratically and has attempted to injure both herself and others. She has harmed herself by tying ligatures around her neck since she was a teenager and has recently been using excessive amounts of alcohol and has been in several fights with members of the public whilst intoxicated. Anita has been brought to the unit by the Police and admitted via Section 136 of The Mental Health Act (1983). Anita is very angry upon admission; she does not want to be on the ward and has asked to go home repeatedly. Your colleague has tried to explain that she is currently detained under The Mental Health Act (1983), and so, at this time, she is unable to leave.

- Consider what the impact of being told she is unable to go home might have on Anita.
- Why do you think this?

Anita becomes very agitated; she screams at your colleague to let her go home, and you can see your colleague becoming tense. They say to Anita 'I've already told you that you can't go home' and they walk away from Anita.

- What do you think would be a good next step? What would you do in this situation?

After your colleague walks away, Anita screams and starts scratching at her face with her nails. She is shouting and swearing loudly, and you can see other service users are becoming upset by Anita's behaviour. Some have started shouting back at Anita and calling her names.

- What is your next step now? How would you manage this situation that is clearly escalating?

Some thoughts for how the situation could be managed would be to take Anita to her bedroom or a quiet/low stimuli room to remove her from the situation that is escalating. If moving Anita would not be possible, then asking other staff to assist in removing other service user's from the area would be a good next step. As Anita has just been admitted, we do not have an established therapeutic relationship with her or a risk assessment or care plan that could help us to know how Anita would prefer us to manage the situation. Once in a calmer environment, we would try to speak to Anita and verbally de-escalate the situation. We would express respect and empathy throughout. Anita is clearly upset and frustrated about not being allowed to go home, so we would talk to her about why that was the case and what would happen next. We could try to explore with Anita what had been happening right before her admission as that may be a significant factor in her distress.

After your conversation with Anita, she becomes very tearful and explains that she doesn't want to be away from her sister. When you understand that this is at the heart of Anita's desire to leave, you ask Anita if she would like you to call her sister so that she could come to visit her. Anita agrees to this and is visibly calmer that she may be able to see her sister soon. Anita then states that she is worried about going out into the ward from the quiet room, you reassure her you will stay with her for the time being and suggest getting a drink in the communal areas. Anita agrees and you sit together in the dining room until she feels more confident about being on the ward. You then approach the team for a debrief of the situation, and your colleague is able to express that they started to get frustrated with Anita and were finding it difficult being shouted at, which is why they removed themselves from the situation. You were able to give feedback on your conversation, and the team reflected on how the situation had progressed and been resolved.

There are several points in this case study that the conflict could have been addressed earlier. Anita may not have understood why she had been brought to the unit by the Police or why she wasn't allowed to go home, your colleague began getting frustrated and so could have de-escalated the conversation about being able to leave more effectively. Anita had a key reason she was so upset, so being able to have a conversation with her and establish how she was thinking and feeling enabled you to make her feel more comfortable and started the development of a therapeutic relationship.

Activity

Think about your clinical area and take some time to consider what could cause frustrations for individuals in your care. These could include factors such as the following:

- Their freedom being restricted.
- Not being able to do things they normally would.
- Being woken up through the night or early in the morning.
- A light being shone through their door throughout the night when they are sleeping.
- Not being able to eat the food they normally like to eat.
- Being around people they don't know or possibly don't like.
- Not having control of the TV.
- Not being able to play games or exercise like they normally would do.
- Not being able to make a hot drink whenever they want to do.
- Having items removed from them, such as chargers which means that they can't charge their devices when they want to charge them.
- Staff changing every shift.
- The environment being loud.
- Not seeing friends and family.
- Not seeing pets.

The list is potentially endless, but it is important that we consider the areas that could cause irritation or frustration in our working environment for clients as we can then potentially mitigate where we are able to but be clear, transparent and empathetic where we can't. This can help us to problem solve with clients as well that is a very helpful strategy to avoid and manage conflict. For example, if a client is frustrated that they can't have their charger in their bedroom and so their phone will die, we could suggest that we keep their phone in the office overnight so it is fully charged in the morning for them and then maybe top it up during meal times so that the client doesn't feel the absence of their phone quite so much. Planning ahead can be an excellent mitigation for conflict as, for that client, their phone dying and not being able to message their friends could be a very significant issue that could lead to real distress.

Conflict, of course, is not just about clients and the potential for it to lead to violence, aggression or self-injurious behaviours, but as discussed in the 'Teamwork' chapter, conflict is a key part of all teamworking.

Chapter 11 Conflict

Vignette

I was working on a night shift with another RMN who was also a member of the permanent staff on that assessment unit. It was a busy ward, and night shifts were no exception! There was a young female from another ward who was in seclusion during that night shift and was very distressed. The policy in that unit was that each ward would do an hour of seclusion observation on rotation, so that it didn't leave one ward short-staffed for an entire shift. The Trust policy was that it had to be a registered Nurse who observed seclusion at all times. When it was approaching my ward's turn to take over the seclusion observation, we received a call from the psychiatric liaison team at the general hospital emergency department advising that there was an individual who would need admitting and they were expecting to be arriving within the next hour. This meant that the client being admitted would arrive whilst either my colleague or I was in the seclusion suite, which was obviously not ideal but certainly not unmanageable. Luckily, the rest of the ward was fairly settled so these were our only two real priorities at this time.

For context, I am female, and my colleague is male. The individual in seclusion was female and she had been distressed and had been undressing whilst in seclusion. She was frequently naked and refused to wear clothes or use the blanket to cover herself when staff requested this to maintain her dignity and respect. She had also become very distressed and agitated at several male members of staff and had made multiple accusations towards male members of staff including that they were looking at her inappropriately and that they had touched her in a sexual manner. In all incidents where these allegations were then made, there were several members of staff present, and she had not been touched inappropriately, but this was part of her current distress and agitation.

Because of this, I felt it was more appropriate for me to do the hour of seclusion observation, but my colleague said that he wanted to go. This led to quite a significant argument about the situation, I felt that as we had the opportunity to do so, we should be mindful of the fact that she was frequently stripping naked and have a female observe to maintain dignity and respect as far as possible. I also couldn't understand why he would want to put himself in a situation where there could be an allegation made with no other witnesses. He got upset with me as he felt like I was saying he wasn't professional and that I didn't recognise he was a nurse as well, capable of doing the observations. The conflict did get heated, and I came to realise that it actually wasn't about seclusion, it was about the new admission. Admissions come with a lot of paperwork. As soon as I said that I'd do the seclusion observations and then do the admission paperwork when I came back, he backed down and agreed to that plan.

I was angry, but ultimately, I didn't care about doing the admission paperwork, if he settled the new individual into the ward and made them comfortable, I was fine doing the administrative side. I went and did the seclusion observations; it all went smoothly and when I returned to the ward, I had had a whole hour to reflect on the situation and ultimately, I was very embarrassed that I had gotten so heated to the point where I had had an argument on the ward with a colleague. Luckily, all of the service users were asleep and far enough away that they hadn't heard or observed anything, but still, I was frustrated with myself that I had let the conflict spiral to that point.

I returned to the ward and could see that my colleague immediately tensed up, possibly expecting another argument or an issue, but I approached him and apologised. I told him I was sorry for getting so upset and that it all got so heated but it was just I had a strong opinion that also included trying to protect him, but I had handled the situation badly. He apologised as well for his role, and we moved on and never had an argument or issue again!

As you can see from this example, none of us are perfect or are able to avoid conflict all the time! What is important, though, is trying to identify when others are starting to get upset or agitated and diffusing the situation as early as possible. When we identify that we are having strong feelings or becoming reactive to a situation, then the sensible thing to do is to remove yourself before the situation escalates.

There is a lot of potential for conflict within all mental health services, with clients, carers, family members and colleagues. We need to recognise that it will happen because frustration happens, we can try to identify potential sources of conflict early, but we need to avoid being scared of all conflict as that is when it tends to escalate. When conflict becomes aggressive or violent, we need to use our communication and de-escalation skills to avoid restrictive practices where we can and use effective debriefing after each incident to understand if we could have improved our de-escalation or management of the situation and learn from each experience as that is how we grow as practitioners and handle conflict well moving forward. Apologising when we haven't handled conflict well or have become reactive also goes a very long way in resolving conflict not only in the moment but on an ongoing basis.

References

Brenig, D., Gade, P. and Voellm, B. (2023) 'Is mental health staff training in de-escalation techniques effective in reducing violent incidents in forensic psychiatric settings? – A systematic review of the literature', *BMC Psychiatry*, 23(1). doi:10.1186/s12888-023-04714-y.

Department of Health (1983) *The Mental Health Act* available at https://www.legislation.gov.uk/ukpga/1983/20 (Accessed: 29 April 2024).

Gildberg, F.A. et al. (2021) 'Conflict management: A qualitative study of mental health staff's perceptions of factors that may influence conflicts with forensic mental health inpatients', *Archives of Psychiatric Nursing*, 35(5), pp. 407–417. doi:10.1016/j.apnu.2021.06.007.

Hallett, N. and Dickens, G.L. (2015) 'De-Escalation: A survey of clinical staff in a secure mental health inpatient service', *International Journal of Mental Health Nursing*, 24(4), pp. 324–333. doi:10.1111/inm.12136.

National Institute for Health and Clinical Excellent (2015) *Overview: Violence and aggression: Short-term management in mental health, health and community settings: Guidance (2015) NICE*. Available at: https://www.nice.org.uk/guidance/ng10 (Accessed: 30 March 2024).

Price, O. et al. (2018) 'The support-control continuum: An investigation of staff perspectives on factors influencing the success or failure of de-escalation techniques for the management of violence and aggression in mental health settings', *International Journal of Nursing Studies*, 77, pp. 197–206. doi:10.1016/j.ijnurstu.2017.10.002.

Pérez-Toribio, A. et al. (2021) 'Relationship between nurses' use of verbal de-escalation and mechanical restraint in acute inpatient mental health care: A retrospective study', *International Journal of Mental Health Nursing*, 31(2), pp. 339–347. doi:10.1111/inm.12961.

CHAPTER 12

Compassion

The term 'compassion' is used frequently in healthcare – from the aim to provide 'compassionate care' to the importance of 'compassionate leadership' and even 'compassion fatigue' – but the term 'compassion' is not always clear or well understood (Gerace, 2020). Within the literature, the concept of 'alleviating suffering' is frequently associated with compassion (Durkin et al., 2019; Younas and Maddigan, 2019; Gerace, 2020) but this would lead us to the concept that only those who are 'suffering' can be treated with compassion. Whilst this may be a core factor in why people present to health and social care services as they are 'suffering' in some way, it almost automatically excludes us from being compassionate to ourselves or our colleagues, mainly if they are not 'suffering' at that time. We also frequently see compassion as a term being used interchangeably with 'empathy' and 'sympathy'; however, there are notable differences between each term. Compassion is sometimes likened to sympathy in the sense that it is seen as a reactive response (Gerace, 2020); however, where sympathy can cause an emotional reaction of 'oh, I feel bad for you', compassion is more reactive in a productive way of 'how can I help you feel better?'. An important factor in empathy and compassion is taking the other person's perspective into account, and we can do that by imagining ourselves in their position, using our own previous experiences of a similar situation and considering normative reactions and responses, such as feeling upset following a friend/family member's death. If sympathy means 'I feel bad for you', empathy could be characterised as 'I feel bad *with* you', and compassion could be understood as 'I can see you feel bad, how can I make this better for you?'. If we utilise this understanding, it can help us to understand what 'compassion' can look like in practice. For example, compassion includes small acts like making a hot drink for someone (Durkin et al., 2019). That hot drink may not 'cure' whatever the individual is experiencing, but it may make their wait a little more comfortable, and so at that moment, you have made it 'better'. We are frequently in a position in health and social care where we cannot make all suffering go away, but we can do small things to make it better and that is the core of compassionate care.

Thriving in Mental Health Nursing, First Edition. Laura Duncan.
© 2025 John Wiley & Sons Ltd. Published 2025 by John Wiley & Sons Ltd.

Why is compassion so important? It was a key finding within the Francis Report (2013) as a significant aspect that was lacking within areas of the Mid-Staffordshire NHS Foundation Trust at that time. Those of us who were working in health and social care at the time of the inquiry and report, I'm certain all remember some of the horrifying details of what happened and failed to understand how it could have been allowed to happen. One example that has always stayed with me is that patients were left without water for days. Water jugs were placed out of reach of very sick patients, and for many, their conditions worsened, or the dehydration and malnutrition caused their deaths. As a nurse, I find it impossible to understand how nurses and other healthcare professionals could walk by someone and fail to notice or care enough to make sure someone had water. It is so fundamental to providing care to anyone that it is still shocking the prevalence at which it happened. Within the Francis Report (2013), this was seen as clear evidence of the lack of compassion that was endemic in certain wards within The Mid-Staffordshire NHS Trust. Of course, there have always been examples of poor care, but generally speaking, these are isolated incidents or singular individuals, sometimes a whole ward/unit with a poor or toxic culture, but poor care on the scale of Mid-Staffordshire NHS Trust was significant and important. In healthcare education, we refer to The Francis Report (2013) throughout many programmes and in nursing, it is crucial learning; however, we are now more than 10 years post-Francis Report (2013) and it feels as if some of the lessons are being forgotten.

One key recommendation that came after The Francis Report (2013) was 'The 6 C's' (care, compassion, competence, courage, communication and commitment) (NHS England, 2012). I vividly remember when they were first launched and being genuinely quite offended that anyone felt the need to tell me, as a registered nurse, that I had to 'Care'! I thought it was ridiculous because I did care very deeply about all of my clients and colleagues, and that's why it felt ridiculous but now I can recognise why it is so important to highlight these traits, particularly to new members of the profession. It can also help to facilitate discussion around each of 'The 6 C's' (NHS England, 2012) in a reflective manner to identify where we may need to improve our practice or skills. For example, if we felt we were being asked to undertake tasks, we were not 'competent' to do, citing 'The 6 C's' could help us to explain our concerns in a productive and positive manner. If a colleague was struggling with the confidence to raise these concerns, we could encourage them to show 'courage'. Utilising the terminology effectively can also help our senior/manager/colleague to understand the exact nature of our concerns. The release of 'The 6 C's' (NHS England, 2012) led to organisations adopting these values and using the same terminology. Many NHS Trusts aimed to become 'compassionate organisations' and some have achieved this.

Organisations being compassionate to their employees is important because, without this, the structures in place do not support leaders to be compassionate, and without compassionate leadership, you will begin to see care that lacks compassion. Evidence shows consistently that compassion has a significant impact on the quality of care being provided (Turan Kavradım et al., 2022) and compassionate care improves patient outcomes (Younas and Maddigan, 2019) but compassion can become eroded when continuously working in stressful and unsupportive environments (Turan Kavradım et al. 2022), so this further highlights that compassionate organisations and leadership are essential to good quality care.

There are several traits that are associated with compassion including possessing good interpersonal and listening skills (Turan Kavradım et al., 2022), being kind, honest and treating others with respect (Durkin et al., 2019) as well as being able to identify and respond to what is important to clients, recognising them as unique individuals (Tierney et al., 2018). Whether compassion can be taught or learned or if it is an inherent skill that some possess and others do not (Durkin et al., 2019) has been a contentious debate for some time. Although some people do seem to have naturally high levels of compassion and find it easy to work compassionately, it can also be taught and developed (Turan Kavradım et al., 2022) and a key way to do this is through reflection. When working with junior staff or students, we can develop compassion as we can with other affective domain skills. The affective domain is one of the three domains of learning/knowledge (the other two being cognitive and psychomotor) and is most closely related to our attitudes. The affective domain can be challenging in terms of education but there are strategies and approaches that can be helpful. These include reflective activities, role modelling compassionate attitudes and behaviours (Durkin et al., 2019) reviewing clinical experiences, role-playing and scenario-based (Younas and Maddigan, 2019) activities.

With this in mind, complete the activities below to understand your own compassion and how you can develop this:

Activity

- What does 'compassion' mean to you? Think not only of a definition of the term but what it really means to you as an individual practitioner.
- When was the last time you think you demonstrated compassion to a client or someone in your care? What did you identify that led to your actions and what actions did you take?
- When was the last time you think you demonstrated compassion to a peer or colleague? As above, identify what happened to lead to your actions and explore what your actions were that were 'compassionate'.
- Consider whether you think you are as compassionate as you could be. Is this something that comes easily to you or something you feel you have developed or could develop further?
- Think about the last interaction you had with a colleague that was difficult and left you feeling irritated or upset with their actions. If you view this interaction through a 'compassionate lens', do you feel any differently about it?

Come back to these activities in a month and redo them, see if you are developing your compassion each month and by completing them, you will begin to see how you can and have developed your skills in this area.

We have considered what compassion is and how we can develop it, but what happens if we develop 'compassion fatigue'? There are several understandings of what 'compassion fatigue is' and it can be a part of or lead to burnout, but it is generally accepted that witnessing distress on a regular basis can lead to compassion fatigue, which then leads to a decrease in empathy and reduced standards of care (Camenzuli-Chetcuti and Haslam, 2021). Compassion fatigue can also occur when healthcare professionals become frustrated with a perceived inability to lessen the suffering of their clients or simply do not see significant progress during treatment (Camenzuli-Chetcuti and Haslam, 2021). Factors that can increase the risk of a clinician developing compassion fatigue can include a lack of self-care, a lack of social support and difficulty in maintaining appropriate boundaries (Mott and Martin, 2019). The potential consequences of compassion fatigue can have a significant impact beyond the professional's own feelings, including poor clinical judgments, abuse or neglect of clients, negative professional relationships and general irritability (Mott and Martin, 2019) which highlights the importance of recognising compassion fatigue in ourselves and others and taking actions to improve it.

As we have identified, a lack of appropriate boundaries, a lack of self-care and a lack of social support can increase the risk of developing compassion fatigue; these are the areas that we can focus on with ourselves and peers/colleagues to support in protecting against compassion fatigue or recovering from this.

Activity

- Think about your clinical area, what are 'appropriate boundaries' within this area? Each clinical specialism will have a unique client group, which will mean the need for different boundaries. Think about what you would feel is appropriate to share with a client or how you would behave with them. One way to understand if a certain action is not appropriate in terms of boundaries is to think 'would I share this practice with other members of the team?', if the answer is 'no' then it is likely to be inappropriate in one way or another.
- If you saw a colleague breaching one of the boundaries you have noted above, how would you approach this? This links back to 'The 6 C's' and having courage, as it is a difficult conversation to have. If we use the example of 'It is crossing a boundary to share your phone number with a client' and you see a colleague to this, what would you say? How would you inform them that you needed to escalate this to their/your line manager?
- What do you do to 'self-care' and maintain your well-being? This is explored in more detail in the 'self-care and well-being' chapter but it is important to consider here also.
- Do you feel you have adequate social support? Do you feel that there is someone either in or out of your work environment that you can talk to about your feelings? If not, how would you improve this?

Our next consideration is 'compassionate leadership'. We will discuss the theoretical elements of this more in the 'leadership' chapter. I will share a vignette from my own clinical practice of having a compassionate leader and then an example of a not-quite-so-compassionate leader. Generally, I don't believe we learn as much from negative examples as we do from positive but in this instance, there are some key takeaway messages about how our actions can be perceived and affect others.

Vignettes

I was around four months post-qualifying and starting my first 'Band 5' role, and my grandmother was dying of pancreatic cancer. She (and the rest of my family) lived around 250 miles away, and to be so far away when your family is going through a situation like that, is tough. My new ward

Manager had barely known me when I told him the situation and that I was trying to go home to see my grandmother as much as possible, but he was kind and supportive. He clearly approached the situation with compassion and empathy as he suggested that we try and cluster my shifts so that my days off were together, facilitating me to go home for a night or two each week if I wanted to. When my grandmother passed away, again, he was supportive and kind. I remember him calling me to check in when I was at home with my family and he told me not to worry about coming back until I was ready and asking if me or my family needed anything. It may not have felt much to him, but it felt like a lot to me.

It can sometimes be difficult to identify *exactly* what it looks like to be a 'compassionate leader' and so as a 'compare and contrast', this is an example of *un-compassionate* leadership. While on shift on one occasion, I was assaulted by a client who was very unwell at that time. I won't detail the assault itself but I was left in a lot of pain and with significant bruising immediately afterwards. I was on shift with a senior nurse who had failed to listen to me when I had escalated my concerns about the client becoming more unwell and that we needed to try and address that in some manner. There was no debrief, which there should have been, and at no point, was I asked if I was even 'ok' by the senior nurse, which I actually was not. I was really very upset and angry that she had not even asked me if I was alright, let alone if I needed any medical attention or to go home, which she should have done. I am sure my discontent was evident for the rest of the shift, and at one point, she said to me in a very mocking and sarcastic tone 'aw, does somebody need a supervision?' I was absolutely infuriated! She should have genuinely and sincerely offered me supervision immediately after the incident, but instead, she ignored me and then thought it was appropriate to mock me several hours later when I had continued to work in significant amounts of pain.

From these two examples, it is clear to see the differences between a 'compassionate' and an 'un-compassionate' leader. When you care about the wellbeing of your colleagues and team, it is very simple to treat them with kindness and be a supportive leader. If you have not previously considered how you can demonstrate compassion to your colleagues, take some time to think about this. We can all laugh and make jokes with colleagues to lighten the mood, but we need to consider our use of 'humour' carefully. I'm sure if you asked that senior nurse about her behaviour, she wouldn't consider anything wrong in what she had said to me as she probably considered it to be a joke but reading the situation from my perspective as the person who was hurt and injured, her actions seem fairly callous and the way she behaved towards me that day, tarnished my opinion of her significantly. A core aspect of being compassionate is trying to see the other person's view, particularly the person who is suffering. I don't believe she considered my feelings that day, which is why I consider it to be an example of un-compassionate leadership.

So how should that situation have played out if that senior nurse was being compassionate towards me? She certainly wasn't responsible for me being assaulted, but following an incident like that happening, as soon as it was resolved, there should have been:

- An immediate debrief with the whole team, including feedback from all members about their thoughts and feelings regarding the incident. The entire team should have been asked if anyone had been hurt or injured in any manner.
- Myself (and anyone else who may have been injured) should have been spoken to 1:1 and asked if we were physically ok, if any injuries were recorded, and asked if we needed medical attention. They also should have offered for me to go home, considering the seriousness of the assault. Most people will seem/be fine to continue, but this should always be provided if they do not feel able to continue their shift.

- An incident form should have been completed, recording my injuries (this was completed by me after I realised, she had not included my injuries in the original incident form).
- I should have been offered genuine ad hoc supervision to support me emotionally following the incident.
- My supervisor/line manager should have been notified of all of these actions so that they were then able to offer/provide support as needed.

There may also be other trust-based policies in your clinical area to be followed in an unfortunate event such as this so please do ensure you follow those fully.

Hopefully, it is clear how a few small and easy-to-follow steps would have changed my entire perception of that individual and the situation. Feeling unsupported in such an extreme way in this incident had an incredibly negative impact on me and our relationship. I'm certain she has grown as a clinician and leader since that time, and would probably be horrified to learn how she made me feel that day. Asking someone how they are, checking in on them and offering support should be a standard part of our practice when working with colleagues, no matter our role or seniority. We find compassion much easier to develop and express with clients, but it is the exact same skill that we can utilise with our colleagues and peers.

References

Camenzuli-Chetcuti, M.L. and Haslam, M.B. (2021) 'Compassion fatigue and mental health nursing: The final taboo?,' *British Journal of Mental Health Nursing*, 10(4), pp. 1–5. doi:10.12968/bjmh.2021.0027.

Durkin, M., Gurbutt, R. and Carson, J. (2019) 'Stakeholder perspectives of compassion in nursing: The development of the compassion strengths model', *Journal of Advanced Nursing*, 75(11), pp. 2910–2922. doi:10.1111/jan.14134.

Francis, R. (2013) *Report of the Mid Stafforshire NHS Foundation Trust Public Inquiry*. 1st ed. London: Stationary Office, p. 23.

Gerace, A. (2020) 'Roses by other names? Empathy, sympathy, and compassion in mental health nursing', *International Journal of Mental Health Nursing*, 29(4), pp. 736–744. doi:10.1111/inm.12714.

Mott, J. and Martin, L.A. (2019) 'Adverse childhood experiences, self-care, and compassion outcomes in mental health providers working with trauma,' *Journal of Clinical Psychology*, 75(6), pp. 1066–1083. doi:10.1002/jclp.22752.

NHS England (2012) *Introducing the 6CS – NHS england*. Available at: https://www.england.nhs.uk/6cs/wp-content/uploads/sites/25/2015/03/introducing-the-6cs.pdf (Accessed: 15 May 2023).

Tierney, S., Bivins, R. and Seers, K. (2018) 'Compassion in nursing: Solution or stereotype?', *Nursing Inquiry*. doi:10.1111/nin.12271.

Turan Kavradım, S. et al. (2022) '"Compassion is the mainstay of nursing care": A qualitative study on the perception of care and compassion in senior nursing students', *Perspectives in Psychiatric Care*, 58(4), pp. 2353–2362. doi:10.1111/ppc.13067.

Younas, A. and Maddigan, J. (2019) 'Proposing a policy framework for nursing education for fostering compassion in nursing students: A critical review', *Journal of Advanced Nursing*, 75(8), pp. 1621–1636. doi:10.1111/jan.13946.

CHAPTER 13

Maintaining Hope

Hope is a very powerful concept. We may not recognise how important hope is in our everyday lives until we feel its absence. As healthcare professionals, we see the real-world impact of hopelessness in clients who are suicidal in particular, and witnessing true hopelessness is heartbreaking. We live in a time where it feels that hatred, negativity and division are escalating across the world (Thomas, 2017) so feeling hopeful can be incredibly difficult but maintaining and inspiring hope should be seen as a core part of our roles as mental health professionals as hope is integral to the human experience and, in and of itself, is a powerful tool in healing and recovery (Laranjeira and Querido 2022).

Hope is defined as being future-oriented (Yeung et al., 2020) in nature and so is fundamental in a recovery-focussed approach to care. As clinicians, we can inspire hope by being strengths-focussed and helping clients in problem-solving, as well as by working in a manner that dispels stigmatised views rather than reinforcing them (Yeung et al., 2020). Being hopeful has been found to increase well-being and reduce negative emotions (Laranjeira and Querido, 2022) and so should be a core tenet of practice.

In the field of mental health, stigma and discrimination have challenged hopeful and recovery-focused approaches; historically, individuals would be told that if they relapsed, they would be unable to get to the level of wellness they were currently at. This is just fundamentally untrue and is demonstrative of an un-hopeful and coercive style of practice. The underpinning message is 'take your medication and do what we tell you to, or you will never be well'. Even in chronic or serious conditions such as Schizophrenia, we need to ensure that our core belief is that recovery is possible for anyone. Recovery for those with ongoing mental health issues is actually more about maintaining control of their life rather than being symptom free (Jacob, 2015) and so focussing on hope, resilience and independence are the foundations of any recovery-focussed approach.

When working clinically, particularly in acute or inpatient services, it is very easy for your hope to be challenged. We frequently focus on the clients who have multiple readmissions that we may feel aren't recovering or staying well in the way that we would have envisioned. There

Thriving in Mental Health Nursing, First Edition. Laura Duncan.
© 2025 John Wiley & Sons Ltd. Published 2025 by John Wiley & Sons Ltd.

are many reasons this can affect us on an emotional level but it can most certainly make us lose hope. What we rarely focus on is the clients who we worked with once and never saw again. It is very easy to have your perspective shifted because of the way the industry works, we never work with people who are doing amazingly and living their lives in a happy and healthy manner! Those who do recover, become well and stay well will also not access our services again, but the numbers of those who may need support at one point in their life, receive that support, recover and never need mental health services again far outweigh those who need consistent support, in my experience. Remembering this can be an important factor in maintaining a hopeful attitude and approach.

When we reflect on our own lives and experiences, I'm sure most people can recognise a period of time that was particularly difficult or challenging in their life. When you felt at your lowest, did you start to feel better at one point or another? It may have taken a long time but most of us can identify an example of feeling bad or low, then feeling better.

Vignette 1

I have talked about my personal experiences of burnout in the 'burnout' chapter but one of the side effects of burnout for me was experiencing depression and quite severe anxiety for the first time in my life. By the time I actually took some time off work, I was crying almost constantly, vomiting from anxiety and having horrific panic attacks on an almost daily basis. When I look back on those times, I mainly think about how horrible it must have been for my husband to witness just how low and panicked I was. I was actually told by my manager that I needed to go off sick (after crying for an hour at her!) and I honestly don't know how bad I would have allowed it to get if she hadn't told me that (so if you are reading, thank you!). I remember trying really hard to think what I should do and then remembered, I'm a mental health nurse, I know this one! So, I called my GP, cried down the phone, and was signed off for a month (I think they went with a month because I could barely get a word out for sobbing), I accepted the offer of antidepressant medication (the first one prescribed didn't do much for me in terms of mood and the side effects were tough but the second one worked well and really helped me) and I referred myself to therapy. In those initial weeks, with the help and encouragement of a close friend who is also a fabulous mental health nurse, I started to be able to differentiate between the 'logical brain' and the 'emotional brain'. When I panicked about what I was doing or not doing, I could try and use a 'logical brain' and think what advice I would give to someone else in my position. Starting therapy was also very helpful because the counsellor I worked with was incredibly reassuring and very much validated my feelings. She recognised how anxious I was and gave me ways to 'bring myself down' when I was spiralling into a panic attack, like putting my feet in a bowl of ice cubes. It's an extreme thing for someone experiencing mild/moderate anxiety but when you're at that level of constant panic, it can be necessary.

After a couple of weeks, when my anxiety had gone from a 10 to an 8, I was able to start thinking a lot clearer and I decided that I was going to do one positive thing a day. That positive thing could be anything that was a 'healthy' activity. This included self-care activities such as taking a bath, doing a face mask, painting my nails, etc.; doing a workout; going for a walk or seeing a friend. Even if I could only manage 10 minutes of one of these activities, it meant that at the end of the day, I didn't feel like I had just sat crying and panicking all day. Over time, I was able to build these activities up, and getting out in nature for a walk every day, in particular, really started to lift my mood. There is a reason that exercise is the first thing suggested for anyone with low mood or anxiety because it works (and it's evidence-based, not just my experience!).

Fortunately, I don't feel like that anymore and I did recover. I attended therapy for around 4 months until my counsellor told me that she didn't feel like I needed her anymore, and I felt strong enough to go back to work. My new line manager was very supportive and I did quite a prolonged phased return, which I think was actually very helpful. I maintained my 'one positive thing a day' and now I can't imagine ever returning to that headspace again because not only have I recovered, but I also learned the factors that led to that in the first place and I learned tools for how to address those feelings before they build to the place they once did. I'm very mindful of time boundaries and taking leave on a regular basis as these were definitely very significant factors that led to everything becoming too much.

There will always be circumstances that could lead to us struggling with our own mental health, even if we think as professionals we should be/are immune! Recognising that you need help, asking for it and accepting it are the first steps on the road to recovery. I can't predict the future but at this moment in time, I can say that I have fully recovered from anxiety and depression.

Vignette 2

I once worked in a psychiatric intensive care unit (PICU) and because of the nature of the unit, being for individuals who needed a higher level of care or security than acute wards could offer, the clients there were generally very unwell. Because the process was for individuals to be transferred to an acute ward rather than being discharged directly from the PICU, it also became quite difficult to maintain that sense of recovery because in that context, recovery was being ready to transfer to another ward. Now, I can recognise that that is absolutely recovery in that context, but at the time, I think it was lost on me. One client that I worked with on that ward spent quite long periods admitted to PICU, and when he was there, he could be fairly hostile to staff and would generally insult you in a fairly vicious way. I think at the time, we all thought that was just part of his personality and that it was maybe just worse when he was unwell. I remember he had a particularly long admission for several months in PICU before being transferred to an acute ward at one point, but then we didn't see him again for a very long time. One day, the Consultant Psychiatrist for that ward came in and told us a story about how she had been asked to speak at a conference. She told us that when she walked out on stage to the podium, who did she see sat front and centre? The former client, who had been particularly vicious in his insults to her when he was admitted. She said she immediately panicked at what he may say or do during her speech. She gave her speech, and he didn't interrupt at all; she said she was too nervous to look directly at him, so she fixed her gaze to the back of the room. Then came the time for 'Questions and Answers', and his hand immediately shot up. She said she was terrified of what was about to happen; he stood up and someone handed him a microphone. The consultant was certain this was going to be the worst thing anyone had ever said and braced herself. He began speaking, 'I don't really have a question, more of a comment. This lady was my consultant for a long time and I cannot thank her and her team enough for all the care and support they gave to me. She is the most wonderful psychiatrist, and I just wanted to take this opportunity to say thank you'.

When the consultant told us this, we were all absolutely floored. We had never known him to have a positive thing to say, and I think we all realised at that moment that actually everything he would say and do when we had cared for him was actually just because of his illness, and it was not his true personality at all. She spoke to him later and said he was so warm and lovely to speak to. Hearing this, made me really evaluate the way I had thought about recovery and hope, because I hadn't ever really considered that maybe the person we worked with wasn't the true version of him, and even though the whole team had always treated him respectfully and with compassion, I don't think any of us thought he would ever recover to the place he did and be living a happy, healthy and positive life.

Now we have considered some vignettes of recovery to inspire hope, we will focus on how to have those recovery-focussed conversations that support individuals in achieving their goals and aspirations. There are many different recovery models that have been developed and can be utilised effectively, but my personal favourite is 'The Recovery Star' developed by MacKeith and Burns (2010). The Recovery Star focusses on 10 areas of an individual's life:

- Managing mental health
- Self-care
- Living skills
- Social networks
- Work
- Relationships
- Addictive behaviour
- Responsibilities
- Identity and self-esteem
- Trust and hope

For each domain, there is a ladder rated 1–10 that is laid out in the shape of a 10-pointed star. The design of the model is for a clinician and client to sit together and discuss each domain individually. It may be that the client feels they are doing really well in most domains, but there is one that they are struggling with, which then becomes your focus to set goals for in how to improve that domain. For example, if someone feels that their social networks domain is of a rate 2, we can ask, 'how do we raise that to a rate of 5?'. This can help facilitate a discussion around what an improved social network means to that person and what steps they could take to get there. They may love boardgames and so could find a local boardgame café or social group to join where they can play boardgames, for example. Once each domain has been discussed and goals have been set, this enables the individual to identify and focus on what *they* feel is important in *their* life. One of the reasons that I find the Recovery Star a helpful tool is that it is focussed on recovery and implicitly is very hopeful. We can all get to a 10/10 for all domains! It's also designed to be used over an ongoing therapeutic relationship so at the next meeting, we bring it back out and look at each domain again. Has there been any change? If there has been a domain that has improved, amazing! We can really identify that progress in a clear and visual manner that will motivate us to continue. If a domain has decreased, that can help to facilitate a discussion as to why something has happened; What has changed? Using this technique can ensure that our conversations are relevant, focussed and future-orientated throughout our time working with a client. It is also something that can transfer between teams as part of a coordinated transfer of care. It would really help a client who is moving from, for example, Child and Adolescent Mental Health Services (CAMHS) to adult services if there was a visual representation of their recovery needs to help them communicate with a new team in a positive, structured and focussed manner.

Activity

Using the MacKeith and Burns (2010) Recovery Star Domains above, rate your own satisfaction in each domain on a scale of 1 (couldn't be any worse) to 10 (couldn't be any better).

Are you surprised by any of the results? For any domains that are an 8 or less, come up with a goal or target of how you could improve it and give yourself a timeframe in which to do it. If you need some ideas, take a look at the 'Self Care and Well-being' chapter.

One of the greatest challenges to maintaining hope for ourselves and others is negative attitudes. We are frequently exposed to negativity from both ourselves and others. We are often most negative in our own internal monologues so take some time to think about how you really talk to yourself. Would you say to anyone else the things you say to yourself? I know I absolutely would never talk to anyone else the way I talk to and about myself! We are very often telling ourselves that we aren't good enough in one way or another, and it's really very damaging to our self-esteem and sense of hope. Are the people you spend time with very negative? That can have a really significant impact on the way we view the world. Are your colleagues very negative? They may be feeling burned out, under-appreciated, tired, overworked and they are all very valid feelings, but if we are in a negative headspace, then we will not be able to see the good in ourselves and others or maintain hope for our clients. Think about how you could challenge negative thoughts and attitudes in yourself and others in a supportive and kind way.

'Fake it until you make it' is a useful concept when thinking about positive attitudes and being hopeful. If we are conscious of how we are presenting and being positive, recovery-focussed and hopeful for others, they will begin to believe it themselves and then will actually start to feel better and recover, which will, in turn, validate your hopeful attitude, reinforcing it for the next interaction you have. When it comes to hope and positivity, you get out what you put in!

To conclude the chapter, we must always maintain hope for our clients and ourselves, especially when someone is unable to hold that hope for themselves at that time. There are millions of stories of recovery, in our clinical practice, we may not always see recovery in the sense we are expecting, but recovery is taking any step forward, however small.

The Chinese philosopher Lao Tzu famously said, 'A journey of a thousand miles begins with a single step' and this is how we should think of any journey to recovery where we have the privilege of being with someone for that first step.

References

Jacob, K.S. (2015) 'Recovery model of mental illness: A complementary approach to psychiatric care', *Indian Journal of Psychological Medicine*, 37(2), pp. 117–119. doi:10.4103/0253-7176.155605.

Laranjeira, C.A. and Querido, A.I. (2022) 'The multidimensional model of hope as a recovery-focused practice in mental health nursing', *Revista Brasileira de Enfermagem*, 75(Suppl 3). doi:10.1590/0034-7167-2021-0474.

MacKeith, J. and Burns, S. (2010). *The Recovery Star: Organisation Guide*. In *Mental Health Providers Forum*, The Mental Health Providers Forum.

Thomas, S.P. (2017) 'Maintaining hope in a time of hatred', *Issues in Mental Health Nursing*, 38(6), pp. 463–463. doi:10.1080/01612840.2017.1319167.

Yeung, W.S. et al. (2020) 'Igniting and maintaining hope: The voices of people living with mental illness', *Community Mental Health Journal*, 56(6), pp. 1044–1052. doi:10.1007/s10597-020-00557-z.

CHAPTER 14

Self-Care and Well-being

Mental health professionals are well versed in 'wellbeing' and the importance of 'self-care', as we discuss this almost daily with our clients. However, Mental Health professionals tend to put their own mental health needs below that of their clients, friends and family (Dattilio, 2023), which is actually very detrimental to their own health and wellbeing. One of the most frequent sayings you will hear in mental health nursing is 'you can't pour from an empty cup', but why are so many of us, as mental health professionals, reticent to acknowledge our own mental health, wellbeing and self-care needs? Why do we not focus on refilling our cups when we need to? Stress and burnout are prevalent across healthcare services, which can have a negative impact on wellbeing and can also lead to developing mental health issues and significant negative physical impacts as well (van Agteren, Iasiello and Lo, 2018). The complex and stressful nature of the work of Mental Health professionals can have serious and significant negative effects on them, including increased rates of alcohol use, depression, suicidal ideation and anxiety when compared to the general population (Dattilio, 2023), with research suggesting that up to 61% of Mental Health professionals may be exhibiting signs of burnout at any given time and that there is an increased level of compassion fatigue (Dattilio, 2023). The increased rate of compassion fatigue in this cohort of professionals can have a significant impact not only on the quality and standard of work we do but also on individual's personal relationships and ability to be empathetic to themselves (Dattilio, 2023).

One of the reasons that stress and burnout are so prevalent within the Mental Health profession is that, ultimately, a core part of our work is witnessing the suffering and distress of others (Rivera-Kloeppel and Mendenhall, 2023). When we accept that that is actually a very challenging thing to face as part of your core role, perhaps we can be a little more accepting of the need to manage our own wellbeing more proactively. When we also consider that there have been increasing challenges with staffing shortages and working with complex clients (Bernburg, Groneberg and Mache, 2020) and the stress and distress caused by working in health and social care during the coronavirus disease 2019 (COVID-19) pandemic (De Vroege and van den Broek, 2023), we can see how many practitioners' cups have run dry.

Thriving in Mental Health Nursing, First Edition. Laura Duncan.
© 2025 John Wiley & Sons Ltd. Published 2025 by John Wiley & Sons Ltd.

It seems that many Mental Health professionals are generally reticent to acknowledge when their own wellbeing is poor and there are many potential reasons for this including that they are avoiding acknowledging their 'weaknesses' (as they may see it) or vulnerability, they are in denial or worry about how they will be perceived if they do disclose concerns or issues (Dattilio, 2023). I think it is important to acknowledge that for any Mental Health professional, it can be incredibly challenging to ask for help. I believe there are many factors that influence that but ultimately, the consequences of us not acknowledging we may need help or support can be significant. Chronic stress has a negative effect on memory, attention and retention of information, (Bernburg, Groneberg and Mache, 2020) which can significantly increase the risk of errors or mistakes occurring. Poor staff wellbeing has been repeatedly linked to decreased quality of patient care (van Agteren, Iasiello and Lo, 2018) which if we cannot acknowledge the need to support our own wellbeing for ourselves, our friends and family, if we understand and acknowledge that our clients will be negatively impacted if we are not 'ok', then maybe we can start to acknowledge that we should be taking greater care of ourselves. Whichever your motivation, friends, family or being able to provide excellent care, hopefully, as professionals, we can see the importance of engaging with our own well-being needs and that self-care is not selfish. It is actually the most important thing we can do to make sure we are being the best version of ourselves possible.

One thing that all professionals can do is to engage in training about stress management and wellbeing, as training and education for healthcare staff in this area has consistently demonstrated positive results that not only decreased symptoms of low mood, agitation and anxiety but also increased job satisfaction (Bernburg, Groneberg and Mache, 2020). Training that focusses on improving wellbeing and resilience has also been evidenced to improve levels of distress and burnout (van Agteren, Iasiello and Lo, 2018) amongst healthcare professionals and Nurses who undertook mindfulness activities reported less emotional exhaustion and reduced feelings of stress at work (Bernburg, Groneberg and Mache, 2020). Self-care is also identified in the literature as a protective factor against compassion fatigue (Rivera-Kloeppel and Mendenhall, 2023). When we consider this evidence of the importance and protective, restorative nature of self-care, then it highlights how self-care and managing our own wellbeing, should be part of healthcare professional's curricula as with Nurse training in particular, the focus is generally on clinically focussed skills without enough focus on psychosocial coping strategies or self-care (Bernburg, Groneberg and Mache, 2020). Perhaps if we embedded the importance of self-care and wellbeing at the beginning of every health and social care professional's career, we would see significant improvements in levels of stress, burnout and compassion fatigue.

Now we have established that we should all be taking greater care of ourselves, what does that look like? There are many examples of self-care that can be beneficial including engaging in hobbies and enjoyable activities, eating well, exercising, having good sleep hygiene (Rivera-Kloeppel and Mendenhall, 2023) and, ultimately, all of the things we would advise our clients to engage with!

Activities

As we have acknowledged, it can be very challenging for Mental Health Professionals to focus on our own needs, so we will first focus on other professionals!

Imagine your favourite colleague, the person who you really enjoy working with and who makes your working day better, has not seemed quite themselves. Where they are normally really upbeat and happy, they have seemed quiet and withdrawn. When you approach them to ask if they are ok, they become tearful and tell you that no, they are not ok and they don't think they can keep working like this for much longer. When you talk to them further, they tell you that they feel tired all the time and are just generally feeling overwhelmed. They talk to you about how they have been feeling very stressed, but there is nothing that has obviously precipitated that, and they feel foolish for being so upset and crying to you.

Now consider what would be your response and advice to your colleague. Take some notes about the key points you would make with your colleague before moving on.

If I were having this conversation, I'd most likely reassure them that there is nothing foolish about this and that I am glad they felt able to talk to me so openly. I would reassure them that most people will feel like this at one point or another and try to normalise this so that they recognise that this isn't anything to be embarrassed about and that having an emotional response to a stressful and complex role is absolutely normal. I'd then explore what they said a little further; they mentioned that they were always tired, are they sleeping ok? If not, we can talk to them about how even one night of poor sleep can affect your mood, and so, of course, they are struggling right now. I'd then talk to them about what they do outside of work that they enjoy and encourage them to engage with their hobbies or social life more, think about engaging with counselling or additional support of that nature, and ask them whether they'd thought about their sleep hygiene. I'd then reassure them that they can come to me any time, if they need anything or just want to talk and that I'd check in with them regularly.

Talking to a colleague in this way can be difficult because we know that they know the advice we are going to give, but sometimes, as an individual, we need to hear it applied to ourselves. Now, giving a colleague advice and support in this way can be challenging but giving it to ourselves (and taking it!) can be nigh on impossible!

Now think about how you've been feeling recently. How are your stress levels? Rate your stress level on a scale of 1–10 (1 being not at all stressed, 10 being 'I've never felt more stress in my life'). How is your mood? How are your energy levels? Rate both these factors and be honest with yourself. How are you scoring? If someone else told you they were scoring in that way, what would you say to them? You may be feeling great, your mood is bright, you feel well rested and although challenging at times, you love your job and find it satisfying and rewarding. If that is how you are feeling, I would guess that you already have self-care built into your life pretty well and you actively consider your wellbeing, which is excellent! Even if we are doing amazingly, we can always put those protective measures in place to make sure we continue to thrive and enjoy our roles and lives. If you are feeling stressed with low mood and low energy, then you need to take some steps to address this. It can be challenging to be honest with ourselves about how we are feeling, but it is a crucial step in improving our resilience, wellbeing and being a reflective practitioner.

We are going to use the National Health Service's (NHS's) '5 Steps to Well-being' (NHS, 2022) to think about how we can improve our own self-care and well-being.

The first step is 'Connect with other people' (NHS, 2022). Do you spend time with people outside of work? Some people are introverts and don't enjoy being around people all the time; there is absolutely personal choice and preference in each of these steps, but human connection and our relationships are important. Being introverted and being isolated are two very different things, do you have as much social contact and engagement as you need to feel fulfilled and supported? If not, reach out to friends, family or colleagues, and suggest an activity or something that means you spend some quality time with people that you enjoy being around. If we are feeling stressed or low in mood, it can be incredibly challenging to reach out and ask for support or contact as we can fear that we may not be good company, or they don't want to spend time with us but this is our negative inner voice speaking and sometimes we need to ignore that negative internal monologue! If you told your friend or family member that you had worried about reaching out, they'd most likely be shocked and upset that you felt like that as most people want to be there for and support our friends and family. If you feel socially isolated, think about activities that you enjoy. Do you like board games? Are you a fan of arts and crafts? History? Musical Theatre? Whatever your personal passions are, there will be other people who enjoy the same things as you! Find a local group on social media and go along! It can be daunting to meet new people but as an adult, it can be very difficult to make new friends, and so if you feel like that, then so do other people! Engaging in an activity that you enjoy will mean that you already have something in common with the other people there as well, so that's a great step to forming new connections!

Step 2 is 'Be physically active' (NHS, 2022). As Mental Health Professionals, we are all aware of the importance of physical activity, movement and spending time outside for our mental health and wellbeing. It can be challenging when you are not in a routine that already involves activity to get started, though, so set yourself small targets, like sitting outside somewhere for 10 minutes, going on a 15-minute walk, going swimming, etc. Whatever it may be, find something active that you enjoy or take pleasure in and try to incorporate it into every day. The benefits of spending 10 minutes doing something active or physical in some ways are not only positive for our physical and mental health but also can mean we feel a sense of achievement and pride that we have done something positive for ourselves every day.

Step 3 is to 'Learn new skills' (NHS, 2022). Learning new skills helps build not only our knowledge but also our confidence and sense of self-worth. There are lots of things we could do in this arena, and that could include attending training for work, engaging with education to improve our skills formally, etc., as well as developing the skills required for our personal lives. Many people find joy in activities such as cooking, but it can be really daunting and overwhelming if you don't already feel you have skills in this area; there are lots of ways you can build or develop new skills, and using the internet as a resource is an excellent way to do this! You may want to undertake a pottery class or learn a new language, whatever your personal interest is, make a decision that you are going to learn or improve those skills and then do it! A sense of achievement and pride can dramatically improve our wellbeing.

Step 4 is 'Give to others' (NHS, 2022). As health and social care professionals, our daily work is ultimately about 'giving to others' and so I think for our professions, this is one step that we need to think more carefully about. I believe that we should acknowledge the work we do and how we support others more as this would immediately improve our sense of self and well-being. Take some time to consider all of the people who are better off for the work you have done. Think of all of the colleagues you have supported; you should get an incredible sense of pride from the positive work you have done throughout your career. One thing we can do more of is acknowledging this for others, thanking them for what they do for us and others, as this improves general positivity and seeing someone else feel valued and supported by you, and these are really positive motivators for ourselves. Helping friends and family with a task like DIY or moving house, etc. can be a really uplifting thing to do, and fostering a closer bond with the person we are supporting can also improve our connection with a sense of reward and accomplishment.

Step 5 is 'Pay attention to the present moment' (NHS, 2022). Most of us as Mental Health Professionals will recommend mindfulness to our clients, but do you engage with mindfulness yourself? Mindfulness is about being present in the moment, and that can include looking at the nature around you as you go for a walk, listening to bird song, feeling the breeze on your skin, etc. or it can be a more structured mindfulness activity. When we are feeling stressed or overwhelmed, it can be particularly difficult to be mindful or feel able to settle to engage in a mindfulness activity. Start off with one minute of breathing; there are lots of videos online that can help you start with very brief mindfulness activities, and the more you practice, the easier it becomes to engage with. If you are struggling with focussing due to lots of thoughts racing around your head, try something that demands your attention – like listing all the countries in the world. It is difficult, and most people will not be able to list all 195 countries, but trying to do so forces you to concentrate on that task and that task alone, which, in itself, is a form of mindfulness.

Within this chapter, we have considered why mental health professionals, in particular, need to focus on their own self-care and well-being and thought about how we can practically do that. We all know that you 'can't pour from an empty cup' and so hopefully this has prompted you to assess how full your cup is and the best way to refill it and keep it full! As professionals, we provide this advice and guidance to others all the time, but it is ok, necessary and important to follow our own advice.

References

Bernburg, M., Groneberg, D. and Mache, S. (2020) 'Professional training in mental health self-care for nurses starting work in hospital departments', *Work*, 67(3), pp. 583–590. doi:10.3233/wor-203311.

Dattilio, F.M. (2023) 'Why some mental health professionals avoid self-care', *Journal of Consulting and Clinical Psychology*, 91(5), pp. 251–253. doi:10.1037/ccp0000818.

de Vroege, L. and van den Broek, A. (2023) 'Post-pandemic self-reported mental health of mental healthcare professionals in the Netherlands compared to during the pandemic – An online longitudinal follow-up study', *Frontiers in Public Health*, 11. doi:10.3389/fpubh.2023.1221427.

NHS (2022) *5 steps to mental wellbeing, NHS choices*. Available at: https://www.nhs.uk/mental-health/self-help/guides-tools-and-activities/five-steps-to-mental-wellbeing/ (Accessed: 12 September 2023).

Rivera-Kloeppel, B. and Mendenhall, T. (2023) 'Examining the relationship between self-care and compassion fatigue in mental health professionals: A critical review', *Traumatology*, 29(2), pp. 163–173. doi:10.1037/trm0000362.

van Agteren, J., Iasiello, M. and Lo, L. (2018) 'Improving the wellbeing and resilience of health services staff via psychological skills training', *BMC Research Notes*, 11(1). doi:10.1186/s13104-018-4034-x.

CHAPTER 15

Burnout

Burnout is one of the biggest reasons that health and social care professionals leave their jobs or careers and is a significant factor in the current record-level vacancies in the NHS, which, at the time of writing, is around 46,000 nurses (Holmes, 2022). The need for focus on Burnout is made very clear when in the most recent National Health Service (NHS) Staff Survey, 24% of nurses *often* thought about leaving, 40% felt burned out because of work and 52% had felt unwell due to work stress (Holmes, 2022). These are dire figures that show just how bad staff are feeling after the most challenging few years in the history of health and social care. We can't ignore the ongoing impact of the global coronavirus disease 2019 (COVID-19) pandemic on health and social care staff; for many, the intense pressure it created has never left. There is an ongoing concern about the long-term emotional scars the pandemic may leave on healthcare professionals (Maben et al., 2022). Nurses are feeling disillusioned and have low morale; the answer is more nurses, better working conditions and better pay, but how can we retain student nurses when they go into practice and experience these negative attitudes and low morale? It becomes a vicious cycle that leads to less and less staff, poorer working conditions, unsafe staffing levels, more burnout and more people leaving the profession. If we are to see real change, we need to start recognising burnout more effectively and supporting staff so that they either don't experience it in the first place or are able to recover from it.

The term 'burnout' may be misunderstood as simply being 'fed up' with work or experiencing some stress but Burnout is actually an all-encompassing reaction to chronic stress that leads to significant emotional and physical symptoms such as; exhaustion, fatigue, sleep impairment, concentration issues, anxiety and even gastrointestinal issues (Collins and Long, 2003). Burnout is actually a process that develops over a prolonged period of time (Wolotira, 2023) and at its worst, leads to absenteeism, poor work performance, negative attitudes, poor interpersonal relationships and resignation. Most concerningly of all, burnout is associated with an increased risk of hopelessness and suicidal thoughts (Wolotira, 2023) and is likely a key reason that suicide rates are higher amongst healthcare professionals (Maben et al., 2022). It is estimated that

Thriving in Mental Health Nursing, First Edition. Laura Duncan.
© 2025 John Wiley & Sons Ltd. Published 2025 by John Wiley & Sons Ltd.

burnout is present in 40–75% of health and social care professionals (Wolotira, 2023) with nurses (Zhang et al., 2020) and specifically, mental health nurses experiencing the highest rates of burnout (Harris et al., 2020) amongst the clinical professions. There are potential reasons for this, including being directly exposed to distress and trauma as a standard aspect of the role (Mott and Martin, 2019) and not seeing significant progress during the period where a client is in your care in terms of a reduction in their suffering or full recovery (Camenzuli-Chetcuti and Haslam, 2021).

There is also a significant negative impact on patient care as research has shown that clinicians working in inpatient environments may start avoiding clients, become less empathetic and could even be abrasive or flippant towards clients, which are indicators of experiencing vicarious traumatisation or burnout (Clarke, 2008). There is also evidence that burnout increases the rate of serious incidents in practice (Harris et al., 2020), which if not debriefed well, can lead to further negative experiences and perceptions of clinicians, which in turn can worsen their burnout and have further impacts on patient care.

When we consider the severity, pervasiveness and consequence of burnout, it becomes clear that it is important to identify it in ourselves and others and to address it in its earliest iterations. In the following activities and case studies, we will identify the early warning signs of burnout, consider strategies to mitigate burnout at all stages and use a case study to consolidate our understanding in a practical manner.

Activity

Some of the earliest signs of burnout include the following:

- Irritability
- Negativity
- Fatigue
- Exhaustion
- Poor sleep

Take some time to reflect on if you have ever felt like this in relation to your work:

- How did this present in you?
- How did you speak to and interact with others?
- Do you think you performed your duties to your normal standard?
- How did this impact your personal life?

Now consider whether you have ever seen these signs in a colleague. If you were to see these signs:

- How would you approach this?
- Would your approach change if you noticed these signs in a peer, manager or junior member of staff?
- What would you do if you believed someone you line managed or mentored was experiencing burnout?

Now we will consider the more moderate–severe levels of burnout, which can include the following:

- Anger
- Anxiety
- Depression or low mood
- Emotional instability
- Absenteeism
- Poor work performance
- Poor standards of care
- Immune system issues – that is, frequently experiencing coughs and colds
- Gastrointestinal issues
- Panic attacks
- Negative attitude to clients
- Negative attitude to colleagues and teammates

Now consider if you have ever felt like this in your career; if so, reflect on the following:

- When did this occur?
- What was happening at that time?
- How did you manage those feelings?
- Do you feel like you were able to recover?
- What would you do if you felt like you were experiencing those feelings again?

Have you ever seen these signs in a colleague? Consider the following:

- How would you support a colleague who was also a friend who may be experiencing this?
- How would you support a junior colleague or student who may be experiencing this?
- What would you do if it were your line manager or someone in a position of authority?

One of the most significant factors in the recovery from burnout is time, support and resilience. One analogy that I have used with colleagues who are experiencing burnout many times is that being burned out is like falling off a cliff edge. You can see yourself approaching that cliff edge, and you can either take action to move away from the cliff edge or you can go over and have to climb back up. It's much easier to not go over the cliff in the first place than to try and climb back up and some people never will climb back up. Leaving the profession due to burnout is 'not climbing back up' which, when you are staring up at a cliff, is an understandable (and even sometimes sensible) course of action to take. We can (hopefully) all agree that we need to keep ourselves and our colleagues away from the edge of the cliff!

The key question, though, is how do we do that? First and foremost, we need to be mindful of our own emotional well-being. Frequently 'checking in' with yourself and reflection is important as a change in attitude is one of the earliest warning signs that you may be becoming burned out. The next step if you are becoming burned out is self-care and seeking help and support. This may look very different to different people and examples of this may be:

- Engaging in activities that are just for your enjoyment, whatever this may be, take time to do something that is purely for your own pleasure.
- Talking to a loved one about how you are feeling.
- Telling a colleague or manager how you are feeling.
- Taking some leave and having a break from work.

- Managing your boundaries regarding work (more on this in the following discussions in this chapter).
- Contact your work's occupational health service or employee assistance service.
- Undergoing counselling or therapy.

Boundaries are incredibly important; as nurses, we are inherently people who want to help others, and staying late at work once in a while is sometimes unavoidable, consistently working late or not taking breaks is not acceptable and will lead to burnout happening much faster. If you work in an environment where you are consistently working late or beyond your contracted hours, you need to raise this with your line manager. There are two solutions to this problem – either your workload is too high and your management needs to address that or you are not working efficiently and in an organised way. Sometimes, we do need to improve our time management skills and our line manager should be someone who we feel comfortable raising that with to help us. We have all known individuals who spend so much time talking about 'how busy' they are that if they focus on the tasks at hand, they will actually get their work done in a timely manner! If our workload is too high, and if this is for a short period (i.e. 1 week where there is a deadline or high levels of acuity or colleagues on leave), then your line manager should support you with either being paid overtime for the additional work or claiming 'Time off in lieu' (TOIL). One organisation I worked for was very diligent with working hours and insisted on TOIL being recorded and reclaimed, which had a positive effect on the team as it was recognised that everyone's time is valuable. We may be inadvertently negatively impacting other's workloads also, particularly by sending emails out-of-hours so time boundaries are a whole team consideration.

Mental health professionals seem to have a particularly hard time in accepting when their mental health may be suffering and that they may need support or intervention. There is an ongoing stigma towards mental health issues that, as mental health professionals, we should be role-modelling healthy attitudes towards disclosure and discussion. There is almost a perception that because we are mental health professionals, we are the experts and should never experience mental health issues ourselves! I have never once had a conversation with a colleague about burnout or that they are feeling exhausted/low/anxious where I haven't thought 'wow, you've been dealing with a lot!'. We hold ourselves to an incredibly high standard, which is ultimately not sustainable when faced with incredible pressure and challenges. One reflective activity that can be helpful when you are not sure what to do about the way you are feeling is to think 'what advice would I give to someone else experiencing this?' and then, however hard it may be to accept, that is probably quite good advice!

When it comes to supporting our team, there are several things that we can do to reduce the negative impact of the work and mitigate against burnout. As colleagues or managers/supervisors, we can ensure we:

- Offer supervision. Supervision is incredibly important in maintaining any clinician's well-being, so there should be a structured supervision arrangement, but all senior members of the team (including those who undertake the 'nurse in charge' role on inpatient wards) should feel comfortable and confident in offering ad hoc supervision also. See 'supervision skills' chapter for detailed guidance and advice in this area.
- De-brief. If there is any negative or difficult incident at work, we need to debrief. Key considerations within a de-brief should be:
  - Is anyone physically hurt or harmed? If so, do they need medical attention or to go home? Forcing a colleague to stay when injured or hurt is deeply inappropriate and will lead to negative thoughts, feelings and attitudes developing.

- Is anyone distressed or upset by the incident? Giving time and space for colleagues to express their thoughts and feelings is vital following a distressing incident. Role model for other members of the team by expressing your thoughts and feelings, particularly if what has occurred was potentially distressing or traumatising.
  - Offer supervision. Some colleagues may not be comfortable expressing their thoughts and feelings in front of the team, so offer to speak with anyone privately if they would prefer that instead.
  - Reflect on what went well and what could have been improved.
  - Listen to any feedback from the team to ensure colleagues feel their opinion is important.
  - Plan what comes next. Allocate someone to check in with the client (if it was a client focussed incident) and to complete any follow-up tasks, such as an incident form.
- Pay attention to our colleagues, has their attitude appeared to change? Do they seem to be behaving differently? Are we worried about them in any way?
- Check in with our colleagues effectively and listen. Ask teammates how they are in a genuine and empathetic way, let them express how they are feeling in a supportive and non-judgmental way and empathise with them. If they are struggling, that does not make them bad nurses; they may just need to take a break or seek some additional support. We do this every day with our clients, but we can extend our skills to support our colleagues as well.
- Escalate your concerns. If you are working in a team where you feel burnout is an issue, raise this with your management. If people are working excessive hours with high caseloads and challenging work, ensure that management knows and if you see poor care standards, you have a duty to escalate this and whistle-blow if necessary.
- Instigate reflective practice if this is not already offered within your workplace. Allowing the team a space to talk together about the challenges and successes of their work can be really powerful in enhancing bonding, building reflective skills and improving service provision.
- Develop resilience together. Reflective practice can be a powerful contributor to developing resilience but there are many other ways of doing this independently and as part of a team. See 'Resilience' chapter for further discussion regarding this.

If we support our colleagues and team effectively and are able to be open and honest about our own thoughts and feelings, including when we are becoming burned out, we will be able to mitigate the negative effects of burnout and 'pull back from the edge of the cliff'. Needing help and support is not a sign of weakness. As mental health professionals, we deal with distressing and traumatising events every day, and this is bound to take a toll on our own mental health at times. Burnout can happen to anyone given enough pressure and stress, and even at its worst, it is recoverable. You can climb back up the cliff and recover from burnout.

Case Study

I have experienced burnout once in my career and unsurprisingly, it was during the pandemic. As with every part of health and social care, my role changed significantly during the pandemic. Many of my colleagues moved to other areas and so ultimately, I went from feeling fairly junior and inexperienced in my role to feeling as though I was the only one left and having to try and run the show as best I could!

There were so many changes happening that had huge sweeping impacts on my work. I constantly had to explain and apologise for things that were so far beyond my control; it was almost laughable! The work that needed doing felt never-ending and I felt I had no one to delegate to. On reflection, there were certainly things I could have delegated but hindsight is 20:20. What this led to was me working 12+ hours per day and working 7 days per week for months on end. Anyone observing this would have been able to predict how that would eventually play out! In my role prior to the pandemic, I probably received about 20 emails a week, and it barely factored into my thinking about my job but as soon as the pandemic hit, I was receiving 300+ emails per day and having almost constant video calls and meetings. This was never how I'd worked or wanted to work. I remember being told by members of my team, on several occasions, that they had been waiting for me to 'go green' on the video calling platform we were using to call me.

I remember clearly that I recognised how I was working was totally unsustainable, but thinking that once we had recruited to all of the vacant roles, it would get better. The realisation that new people couldn't just take on everything; they needed guidance, training and support was devastating.

Burnout will present differently in different people but for me, it presented as crying in the shower every morning and vomiting frequently from anxiety and panic. I felt like I couldn't breathe and that I was having a low-level panic attack all of the time. I knew this wasn't normal while it was happening; of course, it wasn't, but the sense of duty to keep going was overwhelming. My sleep was dire; I was waking up throughout the night and probably averaging about 3 hours a night for around 6 months when it was at its worst.

I would keep working until I couldn't read what was in front of me anymore. I would be logging off at 10 p.m., having cleared my inbox before 6 p.m. and then starting the actual work I needed to do, I would still have 50+ emails when I gave up on sleep and logged back in to start the next day at 6 a.m.

One factor that I came to realise was having an incredibly negative effect was that working from home, I could never 'get away' from my work. I was working in the living room on the dining table and would close my laptop in the evening but still be able to see it when trying to spend time with my partner or watch TV etc.

I stopped being able to retain information and started making mistakes. This is entirely predictable when you are working ridiculous hours and not sleeping. I remember having to ask the same question to a colleague again and again and again. I remember even saying to him 'I know I've asked you this multiple times but I can't retain it'. You would think that would have been the moment I recognised it had gone too far.... But it wasn't!

I carried on, I asked for help but nothing happened that would actually help me. I had new starters, and I tried to support them, but on reflection, they probably felt they had been thrown into the deep end! I eventually got to the point where I took some leave. I could not tell you how many months of crying every day and constant panic had occurred at that point. I actually only took leave then because I was meant to be getting married and had booked it months before! I took 2 weeks off and I still cried every day. I remember thinking throughout that period that 'it's only 9 days before I have to go back', 'it's only 2 days before I have to go back'. I did not switch off or relax at all because I was filled with terror at returning to work.

Monday came and I did return to work. A colleague told me later that they had spoken to me that day and knew I wasn't ok, I seemed flat and disconnected. I had a meeting with my line manager on a Tuesday morning about an unrelated matter, and as soon as she asked me how I was, I started sobbing and couldn't stop. I'd gone over the cliff edge.

My manager told me to close my laptop and walk away from it. She told me to call my GP and get signed off sick. I didn't argue with her because I couldn't. I felt utterly broken. I have never felt that level of despair or panic in my life; I have never been that low, but I needed someone to tell me to go off sick.

The days after that were consumed by guilt. I felt awful for letting people down; I felt ridiculous for being in the state I was and that I shouldn't feel like this, I needed to pull myself together! I went to see a very close friend in the days after and nearly turned around several times because I couldn't stop crying in the car and thought she would hate me for going over and being such poor company. She was wonderful (she is also a Mental Health Nurse who I trained and worked with) and said everything I needed to hear in that moment. Particularly, that no one could have sustained what I had without being affected by it. She also made me reflect on what I would say to anyone else feeling the way I was and this became such a powerful tool in my recovery from burnout.

I did what I would advise others to do: I spoke to my general physician (GP), I found a therapist and I did what they suggested. I also stopped punishing myself for being burned out. It took 4 months, but I felt better; I did climb back up the cliff (thank you to therapy in particular for that one!) and I returned to work. I had a new line manager at this point who was incredibly supportive and protective of me moving forward. I did a phased return and then used leave to take regular breaks. I take regular leave now, and I am incredibly time-bound. I do not work beyond my contracted hours unless there is something very time-sensitive and important, and on those occasions, I reclaim that time as TOIL.

I promised myself and my husband that I would never get to that place again; hitting burnout (which I only named after about a month of therapy!) is an awful feeling. It truly is all-encompassing. If you are feeling that way though, please learn from my example and steer away from the edge of the cliff! Taking 1 week of leave when you are starting to feel burned out is much more effective and efficient than taking months off to recover from full burnout. If you can't do it for yourself, do it for your loved ones, clients and team. You are irreplaceable to your family, but your work will always get covered in one way or another so if you take one thing from this chapter, it's the importance of you and your wellbeing.

References

Camenzuli-Chetcuti, M.L. and Haslam, M.B. (2021) 'Compassion fatigue and mental health nursing: The final taboo?,' *British Journal of Mental Health Nursing*, 10(4), pp. 1–5. doi:10.12968/bjmh.2021.0027.

Clarke, V. (2008) 'Working with survivors of trauma,' *Mental Health Practice*, 11(7), pp. 14–17. doi:10.7748/mhp2008.04.11.7.14.c6481.

Collins, S. and Long, A. (2003) 'Working with the psychological effects of trauma: Consequences for mental healthcare workers – A literature review,' *Journal of Psychiatric and Mental Health Nursing*, 10(4), pp. 417–424. doi:10.1046/j.1365-2850.2003.00620.x.

Harris, O. et al. (2020) 'Surviving and thriving – A mixed-methods study of staff experiences of occupational wellbeing in a psychiatric place of safety service,' *Journal of Mental Health*, 32(1), pp. 158–165. doi:10.1080/09638237.2020.1844870.

Holmes, J. (2022) *The NHS nursing workforce – have the floodgates opened?, The King's Fund*. Available at: https://www.kingsfund.org.uk/blog/2022/10/nhs-nursing-workforce#:~:text=Over%20the%20past%2012%20months,cent%20on%20the%20previous%20year (Accessed: 21 April 2023).

Maben, J. et al. (2022) '"You can't walk through water without getting wet" UK nurses' distress and psychological health needs during the COVID-19 pandemic: A longitudinal interview study,' *International Journal of Nursing Studies*, 131, p. 104242. doi:10.1016/j.ijnurstu.2022.104242.

Mott, J. and Martin, L.A. (2019) 'Adverse childhood experiences, self-care, and compassion outcomes in mental health providers working with trauma,' *Journal of Clinical Psychology*, 75(6), pp. 1066–1083. doi:10.1002/jclp.22752.

Wolotira, E.A. (2023) 'Trauma, compassion fatigue, and burnout in nurses,' *Nurse Leader*, 21(2), pp. 202–206. doi:10.1016/j.mnl.2022.04.009.

Zhang, X.J. et al. (2020) 'Interventions to reduce burnout of physicians and nurses,' *Medicine*, 99(26). doi:10.1097/md.0000000000020992.

CHAPTER 16

Stigma and Discrimination

Stigma and discrimination could be argued to be one of the most important and significant issues in the field of mental health. The impact it has on individuals and on the wider society cannot be overstated, and it is something that all of us can work to improve in small and big ways. There are many definitions of stigma and many types of stigma that will be explored, but ultimately, stigma can be defined as negative stereotypes/attitudes that can lead to discrimination (Pinfold, Byrne and Toulmin, 2005). When someone is treated unfairly or differently due to an attribute that they have (or are perceived to have), such as having a mental health issue, this is what we would define as discrimination (Jeffrey et al., 2013). Knowledge, attitude and behaviour are all interconnected and ultimately relate to ignorance, prejudice and discrimination (Thornicroft et al., 2016). Stigma and discrimination can affect access to care and support not only on an individual level but on an institutional and community level as well through lack of service provision and poor funding to negative attitudes about accessing mental health care (Henderson, Evans-Lacko and Thornicroft, 2013).

So where does stigma come from? Ultimately, stigma comes from negative stereotypes, which are beliefs about a group of people (Thornicroft et al., 2016). We don't necessarily believe stereotypes, even if we are aware of them, but when we do believe in them, and they provoke negative emotional reactions, this is when it becomes prejudice (Kaushik, Kostaki and Kyriakopoulos, 2016). Prejudice usually leads to avoidance and distancing, which then means the stigmatised person or group are then experiencing discrimination as they are being avoided or excluded specifically because of a characteristic they hold (Kaushik, Kostaki and Kyriakopoulos, 2016), that usually they have no control over or choice about. Stereotypes and prejudice expressed by individuals or a society-held view are defined as 'public stigma'; 'structural stigma' is where laws or policies enact discrimination (Henderson and Gronholm, 2018). 'Courtesy stigma' is where someone who has an association with a member of a stigmatised group is stigmatised by association, 'provider-based stigma' is when it is experienced by professionals who should be providing assistance, and 'self-stigma' is when people believe the publicly held negative beliefs and apply them to themselves (Henderson and Gronholm, 2018). Not everyone who experiences

Thriving in Mental Health Nursing, First Edition. Laura Duncan.
© 2025 John Wiley & Sons Ltd. Published 2025 by John Wiley & Sons Ltd.

mental health issues will experience self-stigma, but for the individuals who do, it is generally understood to lower self-esteem and cause a worsening of mood (Bowen, 2016) as well as a significant fear of rejection (Quinn, Williams and Weisz, 2015) that can impact all social aspects of an individual's life.

There are a lot of different terms used within any discussion of stigma and discrimination but it can be difficult to understand what each term/definition would look like in real life. To address this, please read through each case study to understand the real-world impact and consider how each could be addressed:

Public Stigma Case Study

Josh is going to a party with his friends for Halloween and has decided to go as a 'psycho killer'. He buys a costume that has a strait-jacket and mask. At the party, lots of his friends think it's hilarious and call him 'psycho Josh' all night, many comment on how scary he looks.

Think about the message this would send. The word 'psycho' is derived from the clinical terms of psychotic or psychopath. Real people experience psychosis and (more rarely) psychopathy. This type of 'costume' feeds into the negative public stereotype that people with mental health issues are dangerous, violent and ultimately something to be feared. Believing that stereotype leads people to be frightened of and avoid people with mental health issues.

Consider if you were friends with Josh and he told you before the party what he was planning to wear, and you understood how this would perpetuate public stigma, what would you say to him? How would you explain that there may be better options? He could dress as 'Hannibal Lecter' if he wants to as that's a character from books and film but using the word 'psycho' as part of and to explain his costume is where the real issue lies.

Structural Stigma Case Study

Amina has experienced psychosis, and was hospitalised, and detained under The Mental Health Act (1983) 5 years ago. Amina has been saving up to go on holiday with her friends to a country that requires evidence of travel insurance to obtain a visa. Amina has tried to buy travel insurance, but she has been refused by several companies, and those who have accepted her have refused to provide coverage in the event she requires mental health care whilst travelling or is charging her more than the holiday would cost for coverage. Amina has decided that she cannot afford to go on holiday with her friends now.

This is an example of structural stigma as travel insurers are private companies with no obligation to provide coverage to anyone, which means that, ultimately, they can refuse coverage or raise the premium for any reason, including historic mental health issues.

If you were Amina's friend, what would you say or do in this scenario?

Courtesy Stigma

Mohammed is 14 and has been struggling at school. His mum has mental health issues and physical health needs, so he does all the shopping, cooking and cleaning at home. He often struggles to get all of his homework done and is always very tired. His friends have started being mean and rude to Mohammed because he doesn't want to spend time with them outside of school because he has lots to do at home and is very tired. They have started taunting Mohammed for his 'crazy mum' and making comments about her and her experiences that Mohammed finds very upsetting.

This is an example of 'courtesy stigma' as the rude comments and offensive behaviour are actually because of a negative perception of his mum, not Mohammed. If you had witnessed the way Mohammed was being treated, what would you say or do? How would you try and support Mohammed?

Provider-Based Stigma

Lucy has a diagnosis of personality disorder and has been admitted to a mental health unit following a period of crisis. Lucy has been injuring herself by scratching and cutting at her skin and feels a compulsion to do so whenever she finds anything sharp that she knows will damage her skin. She doesn't really know why she feels like this but feels relief from the experience of pain. She found a stone outside in the ward garden, put it in her pocket and went back to her bedroom, where she began scratching herself with the stone. One of the staff came past and noticed what Lucy was doing. She shouted for other staff and they attended and took the stone off Lucy. They asked her why she had been scratching herself and Lucy responded 'I don't know'. The staff member rolled their eyes and started to walk out of the room. As they did, they said to the other staff member 'This is why I hate working with PDs, they're always doing something attention seeking'.

In this example, you can see that the staff member has a negative and stigmatised attitude, specifically towards clients with a diagnosis of Personality Disorder. If you witnessed a colleague making statements like this, what would you do? How would you react? What impact do you think attitudes such as this have on the delivery of care? Do you think Lucy is receiving the highest standards of care possible?

Self-Stigma Case Study

Sylvester has been under a lot of pressure at work recently and has been working increasingly long hours to try and keep up. He began worrying more and more about work issues, then he started having difficulties sleeping. He found he couldn't stop worrying about work when he tried to go to bed and would frequently wake up in the night panicking about how much he had to do the next day. He has started to feel that he can't cope or keep up any longer and he would panic about losing his job. After several months of not sleeping, he decided to go to his GP to ask for medication to help him sleep. When he told the doctor how he had been feeling and why he was struggling to sleep, the doctor suggested that he thought Sylvester may have generalised anxiety disorder and that talking therapies and some time off work could help him. Sylvester was shocked as he had never thought he had anxiety. Following the appointment, Sylvester did not want to go to talking therapies or seek professional help. Sylvester also didn't want to take any time off work or disclose his new diagnosis as he thought his boss and team would think he was 'weak'. Sylvester stopped spending time with his friends and engaging in activities he normally enjoyed, like going to the cinema and paddleboarding, because he thought 'someone with anxiety' shouldn't do those things and he didn't want anyone to find out. Sylvester stayed at home, alone almost all of the time for fear of anyone knowing how he had been feeling because he thought he would be judged by his friends who wouldn't want to know him anymore.

In this example, you can see how having a negative perception of an individual with anxiety became damaging because this was then something that Sylvester applied to himself. If you were friends with Sylvester and he suddenly stopped attending activities, how would you approach this? What if Sylvester expressed this was how he was feeling? How would you reassure him or encourage him to seek help? How would you support him in disclosing his condition and concerns to his employer?

As we can see, there are multiple facets to stigma (Henderson and Gronholm, 2018) including whether it is perceived (which may be a belief that many people hold), endorsed (agreement with the negative belief), anticipated (the individual holds that belief so believes others will if they have that characteristic), received (expressed negativity in relation to the characteristic) or enacted (discrimination – like denying a job). Now we have considered the types of stigma and how they may present, let's consider discrimination. As we have mentioned, discrimination is effectively the active effect of stigma. If stigma is related to your thoughts and feelings, discrimination is related to your actions. Discrimination can be very subtle but it can also be very severe and have significant ramifications. Those who experience more discrimination have higher levels of self-stigma (Quinn, Williams and Weisz, 2015), which, as already discussed, impacts an individual and their life in a myriad of negative ways. Having a mental health diagnosis has been found to lead to reduced access to employment opportunities, being more likely to experience poverty, and fewer social networks (Pinfold, Byrne and Toulmin, 2005). The majority of individuals with a mental health diagnosis will avoid disclosure, particularly to potential employers or may even not apply for a role due to the fear of being discriminated against or the feeling that it is inevitable if they were to disclose (Pinfold, Byrne and Toulmin, 2005). This fear appears to be valid as research has shown clearly that those who are in a position to employ others will not extend the same opportunities to those who disclose mental health issues in comparison with those who do not (Henderson and Gronholm, 2018). This could mean not offering a job in the first place or denying progression opportunities such as training or promotions. Clearly, not all individuals who are in a position to employ others hold negative beliefs or stereotypes regarding those with mental health issues, and many individuals actively want to support their employees or junior members of the team. Managers/leaders who are openly positive and proactive about mental health issues can have a very positive effect, as research has shown that how supportive a manager is perceived to be has a significant impact on whether an employee will feel able to disclose a mental health issue (Waugh et al., 2017).

Discrimination does not just affect employment opportunities, which is obviously a significant area on its own, but it is much more pervasive and far-reaching. Stigma and discrimination affect individuals in a multitude of arenas when they experience mental health issues and this includes being the target of violence, abuse, sexual or financial exploitation, education, the criminal justice system, care and housing (Henderson and Gronholm, 2018). Research has found that individuals with mental health issues who have children are perceived as bad parents (Jeffrey et al., 2013) and that there is a distinct lack of support for parents with mental health issues in terms of how-to parent well and effectively. In Jeffrey et al.'s (2013) study, there were deeply disturbing findings including that parents with mental health issues were given poor or incorrect family planning and mental health management advice. This included falsehoods such as that 'no medication can be taken during pregnancy', leading to individuals believing they will become unwell or relapse if they choose to start a family – which is factually incorrect as many mental health medications are believed to be safe in pregnancy and during breastfeeding, specialist advice from Perinatal Mental Health Teams should be sought to ensure that parent and baby are supported appropriately. Respondents to the Jeffrey et al. study (2013) also reported that they frequently experienced provider-based stigma and felt that professionals involved in their care (including maternity services, mental health services, emergency services and social workers) did not believe they were safe or trustworthy parents. The ramifications of feeling this way about health and social care providers can be incredibly serious and significant. A parent who believes they will be judged in this way is likely to avoid services, even if they want to ask for help. The potential impact on children in this scenario is deeply concerning as they may then be denied help, care and treatment that could benefit them and help them to thrive purely because the parent fears judgment and discrimination.

When you consider the impact of these two areas in particular, employment opportunities (which ultimately determines financial stability and lifestyle) and family planning, it becomes clearer why addressing stigma and discrimination is so vitally important. It has also been found that the consequence of stigma and discrimination can actually make an individual's mental health worse (Thornicroft et al., 2016). It also highlights how addressing stigma and discrimination is the responsibility of everyone, particularly health and social care professionals.

Provider-based discrimination is possibly one of the most puzzling concepts. It is frequently cited in literature that the attitudes and perceptions of healthcare professionals (which includes mental health professionals of all disciplines) are a significant source of stigma, negative attitudes and discrimination (Thornicroft et al., 2016) but not only that, perceived discrimination or negative attitudes has been found to increase the risk of suicidal thoughts or attempts. This is quite literally the opposite of what healthcare professionals are meant to do! One of the most stigmatised conditions is personality disorder with many mental health professionals feeling that they are poorly equipped to work with clients with this diagnosis and individuals experiencing personality disorder feel that some staff demonstrates prejudicial attitudes and that they are frequently excluded from, or provided with poorer levels of care and service (Bowen, 2016). In healthcare literature, the diagnosis of personality disorder is frequently labelled as 'difficult', which further highlights the pervasive nature of stigma amongst healthcare professionals (Clark et al., 2014). One of the most significant barriers to individuals seeking help, care and support is negative experiences with healthcare professionals from all specialisms (Henderson, Evans-Lacko and Thornicroft, 2013). Many individuals with mental health issues report that they have been treated disrespectfully, experienced worse waiting times and have been treated as though their physical health issues are imagined by healthcare staff (Waugh et al., 2017). Negative attitudes towards clients do not just affect the client group, though, as research has found that professionals who hold stigmatised views of certain client groups are also more likely to experience burnout and poorer general health themselves (Clark et al., 2014). This does not have to continue to be the case though. Even brief training interventions focussing on knowledge, understanding and attitudes to clients with a diagnosis of personality disorder were found to have significant benefits that were sustained (Clark et al., 2014), which highlights the need for training and education that focusses on not only knowledge and understanding but also attitude. I believe one of the reasons that healthcare professionals hold stigmatised beliefs regarding clients with a diagnosis of Personality Disorder specifically is due to poor understanding of the condition. Battle et al. (2004) found that of individuals who were diagnosed with borderline personality disorder, 82% had experienced childhood neglect, 73% had experienced childhood abuse and 44% experienced childhood sexual abuse. If we reframed our understanding of Personality Disorder to be caused by complex trauma during childhood and adolescence, then perhaps clinicians would be more inclined to treat people with greater compassion and empathy.

Stigma and discrimination, of course, do not just exist from healthcare professionals, stigmatised attitudes exist in wider society, and generally, the negative and prejudicial perceptions of individuals with mental health issues are largely due to mental health being very poorly understood by the general population (Waugh et al., 2017). One of the most concerning effects of stigma is that it has a negative effect on seeking help and support (Clement et al., 2014) with estimates of up to 74% of individuals experiencing symptoms of mental health issues not receiving treatment. Many people avoid seeking care because they don't understand that there is treatment and support available that does work for the majority of people (Henderson, Evans-Lacko and Thornicroft, 2013). Delays in treatment of conditions, such as psychosis, schizophrenia, bipolar affective disorder and anxiety disorders, are linked to poorer outcomes (Clement et al., 2014) which highlights the importance of raising public awareness of what mental health issues are and what support is available to them. There have been a number of campaigns within the UK to try and improve public knowledge and attitudes such as 'Time to Change' and research suggests that increased knowledge and understanding about mental health i.e. improving mental health literacy, increases the likelihood of someone disclosing to friends or family their concerns and going on to receive some form of support (Henderson, Evans-Lacko and Thornicroft, 2013). There have, however, been a number of campaigns targeted at improving knowledge and attitudes towards mental health, and research suggests the overall impact of mass media interventions on stigma and discrimination is unclear and inconsistent, with some campaigns having only identified marginal reductions in discrimination or prejudice (Clement et al., 2013). The reason for the inconsistency in the literature may be due to the focus of these campaigns. Many of these campaigns focus on symptoms of anxiety and depression in particular, which is obviously needed and necessary as these are the most common mental health conditions that many people will experience at one point in their lives. These campaigns however rarely mention other mental health conditions such as schizophrenia, psychosis, bipolar affective disorder, post-traumatic stress disorder, Eating Disorders or Personality Disorder and so where they have likely had a positive impact on those feeling low in mood or experiencing anxiety feel better able to disclose their thoughts and feelings to friends, family or professionals for support, other conditions are still rarely discussed and poorly understood by the general population. As mass media campaigns can be a force for change and improvement, it can also be incredibly detrimental. Historically, media representations of mental health issues have been very negative, and research has found the majority of media representations of mental health tend to sensationalist violence and danger, which increases the stigmatised view that those with mental health issues are violent or dangerous (Bowen 2016). An example of this is that an analysis of British tabloid newspapers showed that these newspapers linked personality disorder to homicide in 42% of articles featuring personality disorders as a subject (Bowen 2016). Considering over 2 million people in the UK will have a diagnosis of personality disorder, it is not representative that 42% of media representations in this context link the diagnosis to murder.

When we consider that one in six people will have experienced symptoms of a common mental health issue *in the past week alone* (Baker and Kirk-Wade, 2023) it highlights the incredible prevalence of mental health issues in everyday life. 20% of the UK population have experienced symptoms of mental health issues in the past week, which really is incredibly significant as a number. Approximately 50% of all mental health issues are evident before the age of 14 (Kaushik, Kostaki and Kyriakopoulous, 2016) which tells us that young people are experiencing this and living with this into adulthood. The statistics regarding young people and mental health are generally very troubling. In an NHS review of data, Newlove-Delgado et al. (2022) reported that:

- 18% of children aged 7–16 years and 22% of young people aged 17–24 years had a probable mental health issue.
- Rates of mental health issues in those aged 17–19 have risen from 10.1% in 2017 to 17.7% in 2020 and rose to 25.7% in 2022.

- 11–16-year-old group of the population with mental health issues are 'less likely to feel safe at school', to report enjoying their learning or having a friend they could turn to for support.
- 17–22-year-old group of the population with mental health issues reported a rate of 14.8% who were living in a home that had struggled with not being able to buy enough food or had had to use a food bank compared to 2.1% of their peers not believed to experience a mental health issue.

(Newlove-Delgado et al., 2022)

What these statistics tell us is not only just how common experiencing a mental health issue is but also how significantly it affects young people. When we consider that there are many consequences to having mental health issues at a young age and although with good support and care, these are by no means inevitable, they can lead to poor educational achievement, substance misuse and poorer physical and sexual health (Kaushik, Kostaki and Kyriakopoulos, 2016). Those with mental health issues are more likely to receive poor physical health care and have unequal access to treatment which increases the risk of premature death (Thornicroft et al., 2016). Most seriously and concerningly there is also an increase in morbidity and mortality from suicide and accidental injury (Kaushik, Kostaki and Kyriakopoulos, 2016) for young people experiencing mental health issues. The key to avoiding these negative and, sometimes, fatal outcomes is seeking appropriate support and care when it is first needed. The most significant barrier to anyone reporting that they are experiencing issues with their mental health or well-being, more generally, is stigma and discrimination, and so this highlights just why this is (as previously stated) one of the most serious and significant issues in the field of mental health.

Now we have considered what stigma and discrimination are, how they affect people and just how many people are impacted by them, we need to consider what we can all do to change things and improve this moving forward. These are my own thoughts, suggestions and principles I try to live by. They are not always easy to maintain all the time, and occasionally, we will make mistakes but the key to improving attitudes and doing better is *trying* to do better.

Mind Your Language!

The words we choose to use have power. They shape not only our thoughts but the thoughts and feelings of those around us. In mental health, there is a myriad of negative words and terms that are used in a pejorative manner that perpetuates stereotypes and instil fear. Some of the most commonly used terms/phrases that need to be addressed and challenged, why and how to do so are:

- 'I'm so OCD' – Unless you actually have obsessive compulsive disorder (OCD), you should never make this statement or any other implying you have a mental health condition. OCD is a very serious condition that has a significant impact on the everyday lives of those with the condition. Many believe that OCD only relates to cleanliness or germs and so use this as a way of expressing that they like to have things clean. There is obviously nothing wrong with liking things to be clean and well-ordered, and it may be very stressful if your home or kitchen is not clean to the standard you are comfortable with; however, the actual condition does not just relate to cleanliness and so it is a significant misunderstanding of the condition. Individuals with OCD may find it is focussed on cleanliness, but it can impact almost any area of life. Many individuals with OCD will find it affects other daily activities like how they get dressed, their routine in leaving the house, how they move through the world, etc., and for someone with

OCD if they are unable to complete their routines in the manner they feel they need to, they believe there will be terrible and traumatic consequences. The impact of this can be significant and far-reaching. Some people may have a specific number that needs to be featured, so turning the light switch on and off 17 times precisely, otherwise, something terrible will happen to them or their loved ones. It can be truly exhausting to live with and can make people feel incredibly isolated. If someone uses clinical terminology in this manner, explain to them why it isn't something to make light of how they may not know if someone they are talking to is living with those thoughts, and how referencing it in an inappropriate manner may make them feel.

- 'Committed suicide' – the reason for addressing this term specifically is the word 'committed'. It relates to when taking your own life was considered a criminal offence but also has connotations of 'being committed' to an institution. Trying to take your own life is no longer a criminal offence, but it is an incredibly difficult situation to experience, and if someone has complete or attempted suicide, we need to be mindful of how we discuss this. Any death by suicide is a tragedy and traumatic for anyone involved, and ensuring that we aren't using outdated terms can help, particularly, those who have lost loved ones to suicide in addressing a small aspect of the stigma that has historically surrounded it.

- '...... is so schizophrenic' – Schizophrenia is a serious mental health issue that can affect people throughout their lives. Individuals experiencing Schizophrenia will face challenges throughout their lives and will experience stigma and discrimination in a very real way. Changeable weather is not 'schizophrenic' and it is really offensive to use clinical terminology to describe *the weather*. This is the context I hear it used in most and likening a real and significant mental health issue to a storm or bad weather generally is in poor taste and perpetuates negative stereotypes. As above, we need to always consider how our words and actions would make someone feel and if you knew the person you were talking to had a diagnosis of Schizophrenia, would you still use it in that manner?

- 'They're a psycho' – as previously mentioned in the examples of stigma, the term 'psycho' relates to the clinical terminology of 'psychotic' or 'psychopathic'. Psychosis is, again, a very serious clinical condition. Most people in the general public have very little understanding of what psychosis or psychopathy truly means, and so they have become generally negative terms with pejorative connotations, and 'psycho' is frequently associated with dangerousness, violence or otherwise poor behaviour that isn't factually linked to psychosis.

- 'That's Crazy' – this is used very commonly in conversation to express surprise or shock most frequently but again perpetuates negative stereotypes of mental illness. Labelling people as 'crazy' is a significant factor in stigma and prevents people from seeking help when they have concerns because they fear receiving this label or people thinking they are 'crazy'. Unlike other terms included here, it isn't a clinical term but instead is a pejorative slang term assigned to those believed to have mental health issues.

- '.... Is so bipolar' – this is another legitimate and serious condition. Most people have a fundamental misunderstanding of what bipolar affective disorder truly is and think it basically means mood swings. Again, people relate this to the weather all the time and again, it is inappropriate to do so. Individuals who have bipolar affective disorder will be affected in different ways but will usually experience prolonged periods of depression and mania/hypomania. 'Rapid cycling bipolar' as a clinical definition actually related to having four episodes of depression or mania *within a year*, not a day, week or month. Most individuals with the condition will experience months of severe depression as part of their condition and this can be debilitating. Mania can

cause people to behave in ways and take risks that they normally wouldn't and again, can affect all areas of their lives. As with the others, it is a clinical term that should be reserved only for that use.
- 'That'll get you committed' – this may be a more dated perspective that (hopefully) isn't as prevalent as it once was. It relates to people basically being threatened with mental health services if they misbehave or, in some ways, don't comply with societal norms. The core issue with this kind of statement is that it perpetuates the belief that mental health care and services are somehow punitive and something to be avoided. If we made people feel more comfortable about asking for help when they feel they need it, people would receive care sooner and have more positive outcomes, recover quicker, and stay well longer with less restrictive or serious interventions. Being admitted against your wishes to a mental health unit is a traumatic experience that everyone (including mental health professionals) would prefer to avoid. Someone seeking help from their GP rather than reaching a crisis point would be the preferred scenario for all involved, so making people fear mental health care and services is incredibly damaging.
- 'The men in white coats are coming for you' – As above, this is hopefully a more archaic stereotype that is not as common in modern times. Mental health professionals don't generally wear 'white coats' so it's a false perception anyway! It again relates to people fearing mental health services and professionals, which impacts help-seeking behaviour in a very real and very negative way.
- 'They were in an asylum' – In the UK, there are no more asylums so it is just factually incorrect to state that someone who received inpatient care 'was in an asylum' recently. Asylums were traditionally huge estates where historically poor care and abuse were rampant. They frequently just removed people from society rather than actively providing care and treatment whereas now, most people will never need inpatient care for their mental health, and for those who do, the principle is to provide support in the community and so inpatient stays are reduced to the minimum possibly needed. If someone does need inpatient care, this is usually because they are very unwell and unable to care for themselves or wish to harm themselves and so having 24/7 care for a brief period will help them to be safe and recover more quickly. Shaming people for receiving care that they need is an awful stance to take and if someone needed to spend a week in a general hospital, would it be discussed in the same way?
- '…. is so triggering' – I hear this term used a lot currently and most of the time, it is because people simply don't like something that is happening. 'Triggering' is a term that relates to someone who has experienced significant trauma (usually that is life-threatening or potentially so in nature) and when we consider the term used appropriate in the example of 'Jenny had served in the military in several active war zones. She now has post-traumatic stress disorder and finds loud, sudden noises such as fireworks very triggering as it immediately reminds her of gunfire', we see how it is used inappropriately in common parlance when something is just less than ideal or in some way frustrating.
- '…. is a PD/schizophrenic/depressive' – this relates to person-first language. People are more than their diagnosis, regardless of what that diagnosis is and we would never think it appropriate to refer to people purely as their diagnosis in other contexts. Someone may have a diagnosis of schizophrenia, etc. but we refer to them as an individual 'with x, y, z' or 'with a diagnosis of …', never just by their diagnosis as that minimises and disregards everything else about them. Just take a second to imagine if you had a diagnosis of this nature, how it would make you feel if that's all anyone ever referred to you as.

Be Kind, Always

This should hopefully be fairly obvious but you never know what someone is struggling with or how they feel. Being kind, approachable and supportive of people will have much further reaches and ramifications than we could ever know. If we show kindness and acceptance to all, all the time in our personal and professional lives then people will ultimately see us as a 'safe space' and so if they are struggling or worried about their mental health, if they feel they can discuss and disclose this to you then ultimately, you could save a life.

Challenge Others

We see poor attitudes, poor care, stigma and discrimination all around us. It can be incredibly hard to speak up and challenge others, but if we do so, then we will be doing one of the *big things* to challenge stigma. If you hear or see a colleague speaking or treating someone else poorly because they have mental health issues (or for any reason), then you need to speak up. We can do this privately, calmly and kindly, but we should always do this when we see or hear stigma and discrimination.

We started this chapter thinking about the big and small things we can ado to address the incredibly significant area of stigma and discrimination. Hopefully, now, at the end of this chapter, you will have a greater understanding of why it happens, what it can look like, and how you can be a positive force to challenge and address stigma and discrimination in the world.

References

Baker, C. and Kirk-Wade, E. (2023) *Mental health statistics: Prevalence, services and funding in England* ... Available at: https://commonslibrary.parliament.uk/research-briefings/sn06988/ (Accessed: 20 July 2023).

Battle, C.L. et al. (2004) 'Childhood maltreatment associated with adult personality disorders: Findings from the collaborative longitudinal personality disorders study', *Journal of Personality Disorders*, 18(2), pp. 193–211. doi:10.1521/pedi.18.2.193.32777.

Bowen, M.L. (2016) 'Stigma: Content analysis of the representation of people with personality disorder in the UK popular press, 2001-2012', *International Journal of Mental Health Nursing*, 25(6), pp. 598–605. doi:10.1111/inm.12213.

Clarke, S. et al. (2014) 'Ameliorating patient stigma amongst staff working with personality disorder: Randomized controlled trial of self-management versus skills training', *Behavioural and Cognitive Psychotherapy*, 43(6), pp. 692–704. doi:10.1017/s1352465814000320.

Clement, S. et al. (2013) 'Mass media interventions for reducing mental health-related stigma', *Cochrane Database of Systematic Reviews*, 2013(7). doi:10.1002/14651858.cd009453.pub2.

Clement, S. et al. (2014) 'What is the impact of mental health-related stigma on help-seeking? A systematic review of Quantitative and Qualitative Studies', *Psychological Medicine*, 45(1), pp. 11–27. doi:10.1017/s0033291714000129.

Department of Health (1983) *The Mental Health Act* available at https://www.legislation.gov.uk/ukpga/1983/20 (Accessed 29 April 2024).

Henderson, C. and Gronholm, P. (2018) 'Mental health related stigma as a "wicked problem": The need to address stigma and consider the consequences', *International Journal of Environmental Research and Public Health*, 15(6), p. 1158. doi:10.3390/ijerph15061158.

Henderson, C., Evans-Lacko, S. and Thornicroft, G. (2013) 'Mental illness stigma, help seeking, and public health programs', *American Journal of Public Health*, 103(5), pp. 777–780. doi:10.2105/ajph.2012.301056.

Jeffery, D. et al. (2013) 'Discrimination in relation to parenthood reported by community psychiatric service users in the UK: A framework analysis', *BMC Psychiatry*, 13(1). doi:10.1186/1471-244x-13-120.

Kaushik, A., Kostaki, E. and Kyriakopoulos, M. (2016) 'The stigma of mental illness in children and adolescents: A systematic review', *Psychiatry Research*, 243, pp. 469–494. doi:10.1016/j.psychres.2016.04.042.

Newlove-Delgado, T. et al. (2022) *Mental health of children and young people in England, 2022, NHS choices*. Available at: https://digital.nhs.uk/data-and-information/publications/statistical/mental-health-of-children-and-young-people-in-england/2022-follow-up-to-the-2017-survey (Accessed: 20 July 2023).

Pinfold, V., Byrne, P. and Toulmin, H. (2005) 'Challenging stigma and discrimination in communities: A focus group study identifying UK mental health service users' Main Campaign Priorities', *International Journal of Social Psychiatry*, 51(2), pp. 128–138. doi:10.1177/0020764005056760.

Quinn, D.M., Williams, M.K. and Weisz, B.M. (2015) 'From discrimination to internalized mental illness stigma: The mediating roles of anticipated discrimination and anticipated stigma', *Psychiatric Rehabilitation Journal*, 38(2), pp. 103–108. doi:10.1037/prj0000136.

Thornicroft, G. et al. (2016) 'Evidence for effective interventions to reduce mental-health-related stigma and discrimination', *The Lancet*, 387(10023), pp. 1123–1132. doi:10.1016/s0140-6736(15)00298-6.

Waugh, W. et al. (2017) 'Exploring experiences of and attitudes towards mental illness and disclosure amongst health care professionals: A qualitative study', *Journal of Mental Health*, 26(5), pp. 457–463. doi:10.1080/09638237.2017.1322184.

CHAPTER 17

Ethical Practice

In nursing, the term 'ethics' can be alienating or confusing to clinicians as it might seem too 'academic' or philosophical and, therefore, not relevant or necessary to practitioners (Roberts, 2004) in their day-to-day clinical role. The overarching principle for all healthcare professionals however is to create 'more good than bad' (Williams, 2009) and determining what is 'good' or 'bad' is ultimately, an ethical decision or dilemma. Ethical understanding and awareness underpins patient safety and the quality of care provided (Uncu and Güneş, 2021). Ethics apply to all aspects of a clinician's role; however, many nurses are not always able to recognise the underlying ethics in each clinical situation (Milliken and Grace, 2015). In mental health nursing in particular, a solid understanding of ethical principles is crucial as rarely are situations clear or straightforward from an ethical perspective for a multitude of reasons, including the very nature of mental health issues and illnesses themselves and the prevalence of coercive and restrictive practices such as the use of seclusion, detention under the Mental Health Act (Department of Health, 1983 as amended in 2007), forced treatment and lack of autonomy or independence. Mental health services continue to be viewed as paternalistic in nature (Roberts, 2004), which imposes hierarchies or staff knowing better and being in charge/in control of all choices and decisions. Power dynamics are an important ethical consideration in mental health (Salzmann-Erikson, 2018).

Beuchamp and Childress (2001) originally stated in 1979 that there are four key pillars of medical ethics: autonomy, beneficence, non-maleficence and justice. These pillars are generally accepted across the health and social care profession as being relevant and appropriate to all aspects of care. They can generally be understood or simplified as follows:

- Autonomy – We all have the right as human beings to make our own choices and decisions about our lives, and as healthcare professionals, we should support and encourage clients to think and act autonomously to make independent and informed decisions about their life and care.

Thriving in Mental Health Nursing, First Edition. Laura Duncan.
© 2025 John Wiley & Sons Ltd. Published 2025 by John Wiley & Sons Ltd.

- Beneficence – All clinical decisions and actions are done with the intention to 'do good' and help improve the life and experience of the client you are working with.
- Non-maleficence – 'Do no harm' is the summary of non-maleficence; at all times, we should avoid ever intentionally causing pain, distress or worsening of symptoms for someone in our care.
- Justice – All individuals should be treated fairly and equitably. We must uphold all laws and rights at all times and people should be able to access the care and support they are entitled to as healthcare is considered a basic human right (Uncu and Güneş, 2021).

In mental health services, it could be argued that we frequently breach the principle of autonomy by detaining someone against their will or using restrictive practices and this is where we can see that ethical issues are commonplace in nursing (Uncu and Güneş, 2021). Healthcare professionals can be seen to be behaving unethically when they are negligent, careless, disrespectful or demonstrate negative, stigmatising attitudes (Slazmann-Erikson, 2018). Paternalistic approaches are in conflict with principles of autonomy which is the freedom to act and make choices for oneself (Roberts, 2004). So why is it sanctioned or continued that we could breach a pillar of medical ethics such as this? Ultimately, it would come down to the balance of autonomy vs. beneficence. If detaining someone under The Mental Health Act (1983) would mean they can receive care and support that improves their life and health, then it may be the appropriate and ethical decision. Capacity is an important consideration within autonomy, and it is due to capacity that sometimes, a paternalistic approach seems to be more ethical or appropriate; however, it should also be beneficent and non-maleficent (Roberts, 2004). There are many different ethical theories and principles that can be adopted or argued as appropriate in healthcare, but we will focus on the aspects of ethics that are most applicable to clinical practice. When there is a particularly challenging ethical issue, it is important to approach this from a multi-disciplinary team perspective (Milliken and Grace, 2015) as this can ensure that all aspects of the situation are explored in a balanced and considered way.

In health and social care, we apply general policies and principles to clinical practice; each clinical area or specialism will have their own that should be followed by any clinician in that environment. It could be argued that by using 'policies', healthcare is applying a 'deontological' approach to care as the process is the primary focus of deontology as, by following a 'good' process, the outcome should be 'good' (Mandal, Ponnambath and Parija, 2016). Utilitarianism is an ethical system that focusses on the greatest good being the outcome, so the process is less important than the final outcome (Williams, 2009). This can seem a very binary approach, but if policies have been developed in accordance with the four pillars (autonomy, beneficence, non-maleficence and justice), then they should be policies that assist in making ethical and fair clinical decisions that support clinicians in knowing how to approach different scenarios, but there will always be occasions where there is either no policy or no guidance to follow, it does not apply to the specific situation or it can be seen that following that policy in this scenario would lead to a negative or poor outcome. Many people would naturally follow a utilitarianism approach as they would consider the outcome of their action/inaction and 'the ends justify the means', but if your actions are positive and morally sound, then the outcome is also likely to be (Williams, 2009). The need to consider the ethical implications of a decision or choice (i.e. 'is this likely to have a positive outcome?') are therefore important, and ethical considerations should form a key part of nursing education including human rights, ethical dilemmas and patient rights (Uncu and Güneş, 2021) as this will assist clinicians at the beginning of their careers to understand ethical principles and how they apply to their practice from the outset and should assist in developing their 'moral sensitivity'.

The concept of moral sensitivity relates to an individual's ability to be aware of ethical issues, fully consider them and make ethically appropriate choices, and having moral sensitivity is seen as the basis to moral and ethical behaviour (Uncu and Güneş, 2021). Understanding and a good awareness of codes of ethics, such as The Nursing and Midwifery Council (NMC) code (2018), are linked to higher levels of ethical or moral sensitivity in student nurses (Milliken and Grace, 2015). Virtue ethics focusses less on what a person should do in a given situation and more on how they should be in terms of their character and values (Roberts, 2004).

Activity

Take some time to consider the character and values you associate with being a nurse:

- These may include traits such as kindness, respect, trustworthiness, etc.

Now consider, how you would develop these values and traits:

- You could develop these through role-modelling, challenging yourself to be more honest and transparent, reflecting on your current personality traits, etc.

From this activity, it can be understood that although not impossible, changing and developing your character and values is difficult and would take a long time. Certain traits like being 'trustworthy' can be easier to develop as you would simply ensure you are always being honest, reliable and dependable and you could hold yourself accountable to those behaviours; however, earning the respect of those around you would be more challenging as that is a matter of other people's perceptions of you.

There are certain specific ethical issues in mental health services, some of which have been mentioned previously but will be explored in further depth. Coercive practice has been common and prevalent in mental health services (Norvoll and Pederson, 2016). Coercive practices can include detaining someone under The Mental Health Act (1983), therefore depriving them of their liberty and independence, but it could also include the use of seclusion, enhanced observations, physical restraint, enforced treatment (such as rapid tranquilisation) and many others. Coercive measures such as seclusion, rapid tranquilisation and restraining individuals are all ethically problematic, and they can be seen as in opposition to basic caring principles and values (Salzmann-Erikson, 2018). For clarity, in this context, coercive practice and 'coercion' are very different. Coercion involves manipulation of individuals such as telling someone if they want to leave the ward when they are admitted informally, they will be detained under The Mental Health

Act (1983). This is an example of coercion and breaches many ethical principles. Threatening to utilise The Mental Health Act (1983) rather than using it appropriately and in the spirit it is intended is morally and ethically wrong. If someone is admitted informally, they have the right to leave at any time. If there is felt to be a clinical risk if they leave, then an appropriate section of The Mental Health Act (1983) should be used, if they are not felt to be detainable and there is no risk identified, then they must be allowed to leave. There may be a discussion or boundaries put in place, but threatening detention to prevent an individual asking to leave is inappropriate and unethical.

Although detaining someone under The Mental Health Act (1983) could be seen as a coercive practice regardless of context due to there being a lack of choice for the individual detained, feeling safe, listened to and being consulted on their views can counterbalance this restriction (Norvoll and Pederson, 2016). The reasoning for someone being detained is also incredibly important as there should always be an identified risk of harm to themselves or others or of deterioration if they were not admitted. The concept of 'least restrictive' principles is also important: Could the individual receive the care and support they need in the community? Supporting people at the earliest opportunity is vital to prevent further distress or deterioration and is also the most ethical approach to providing care. In their research, Norvoll and Pederson (2016) noted that several participants had reported that they had sought help but didn't receive it until they were then too ill to be able to consent to an inpatient admission or other treatment options. This highlights the importance of community services and teams being able to identify and intervene at the earliest opportunity.

When considering inpatient services in particular, they can be very challenging environments for various reasons (Salzmann-Erikson, 2018), but the rapid and changing nature of an inpatient service can involve situations and scenarios that can become ethically challenging. The balance of maintaining a safe environment can be difficult when also considering individual patient needs (Salzmann-Erikson, 2018). The concept of 'the greater good' can become prominent in these services, and this is particularly apparent for individuals who are detained for long periods of time in higher security environments, such as forensic mental health services. Forensic services have a strong focus on community safety; the long-term detention of an individual is outweighed by the protection of the public, 'the greater good' (Williams, 2009). There are of course considerations that involve agencies outside of health and social care such as The Criminal Justice System in such services and the balance of care vs. community safety and public perception can be difficult to manage. Within inpatient services, there are also concerns regarding violence and aggression and how to manage such issues that can happen frequently. The concept of coercive or restrictive practices when there is legitimate risk of harm to others through violence or aggression has been identified by service users as appropriate and justified; however, the antecedents to violent or aggressive behaviour need to be identified and addressed appropriately as the trigger for violence could well be the inpatient environment itself (Norvoll and Pederson, 2016). Violence and aggression in inpatient services are usually seen as purely about the service user and their characteristics, but this does not take into account the nature of the ward and staff that may actually be the root cause for violence or aggression (Salzmann-Erikson, 2018). Studies have found that nurses link violence to being unwell, whereas service users link violence to poor communication from staff (Salzmann-Erikson, 2018). There will always be occasions where restrictive practices such as the use of restraint, seclusion or rapid tranquilisation will be the ethically appropriate decision to prevent further harm, damage or even death, but restrictive practices such as these must always be proportionate and purposeful (Norvoll and Pederson, 2016).

Case Study

As discussed above, ethics can feel alienating or irrelevant to clinical practice, so the below case study is intended to help link the core principles of ethics to real-world scenarios. This may seem an extreme example; however, this is based on a real situation that occurred.

Mrs T is a 64-year-old female who has been admitted to your ward. She has been brought to the ward with her care co-ordinator (Asha), an Approved Mental Health Practitioner, and accompanied by two police officers as she has been detained under Section 135 of The Mental Health Act (1983). Asha informs you that it has been several weeks since she was able to have any contact with Mrs T despite multiple attempts to visit her at home. Asha has worked with Mrs T for several years and knows her well. Asha reports that Mrs T is normally very friendly and engaged and appears to enjoy Asha's visits to her home, but when Mrs T has previously become unwell, she isolates herself and stops having any social contact. Asha's concerns had been growing for some time and worried that Mrs T had become very unwell and had run out of options to engage with her and so applying for a Section 135 warrant was discussed with the Multi-Disciplinary Team (MDT) and it felt to be the most appropriate option to ensure that Mrs T was ok and, if not, to bring her to hospital for care and treatment.

When they attended Mrs T's home, she refused to open the door despite lengthy attempts from Asha, the Approved Mental Health Practitioner (AMHP) and police to communicate with her through the letterbox. It was only when the police advised Mrs T that they would have to force entry to her home that she opened the front door. Asha reported that she was shocked at Mrs T's appearance. She had lost a significant amount of weight, and Mrs T normally took great pride in her appearance but today she appeared dishevelled, in visibly dirty clothes and her hair appeared to have been unwashed for quite some time. Asha was deeply concerned as it was clear that Mrs T had become very unwell and was not caring for herself adequately. Mrs T was also very angry and rude towards Asha, which Asha had never experienced with Mrs T previously.

Once they entered Mrs T's home, Asha could see that the home was also uncared for, where it was normally spotless and beautifully clean. Asha entered the kitchen, whilst the AMHP and police spoke with Mrs T and found there was no food in the cupboards or fridge, and there was no evidence of food in the kitchen bin or outside bin. Asha was deeply concerned that Mrs T had not been eating anything and that this could have been ongoing for several weeks.

Mrs T did not want to speak to any staff after being admitted to the ward, she was shown to her room and welcomed to the ward but told staff she would not speak to them. Several staff approached Mrs T to try and engage with her, but she became more and more irate at them 'bothering' her.

From the handover received from Asha, there were several concerns identified, but the most urgent was that Mrs T had potentially not been eating adequately for several weeks. This raised the possibility of refeeding syndrome. Refeeding syndrome is a clinical condition that can occur in individuals who have had poor/no nutritional intake for several days or weeks. Refeeding syndrome can cause significant physical ramifications and can ultimately be fatal. If someone who has not eaten adequately for some time begins eating a normal diet and full meals again, this can trigger the syndrome and so if it is suspected, a careful diet that slowly builds up to a normal food and fluid intake is imperative. The only way to confirm whether someone is likely to develop refeeding syndrome is to check the blood levels of key indicators such as potassium. The team decides that this is an urgent priority and that blood tests are needed as quickly as possible.

You approach Mrs T to try and explain the situation and concerns to her, but she is unreceptive and refuses to consent to having blood taken.

The ethical dilemma here is:

- Do you (as a team) not persist with the need for a blood test for Mrs T, advise her of the risks and allow her to make a decision as to whether she eats a meal without a blood test?
- Or inform Mrs T that due to the level of risk that if she does not consent to having her blood taken, she will be forcibly restrained so that a blood sample can be taken?

Consider these issues and make a decision as to which option you would advocate for in this scenario. What are the ethical issues you can identify in this scenario?

Outcome

In this scenario (that is based on a true event), after a lengthy team discussion, it was decided that we would continue to try and engage with Mrs T in an attempt to encourage her to willingly consent to bloods whilst restricting her food intake to avoid refeeding syndrome occurring in the interim. One staff member was identified to have developed some rapport with Mrs T and so they were tasked on leading with Mrs T and a timeframe of three hours was set where the ward Doctor would remain available so that if Mrs T were to consent, the blood test could be taken immediately. After three hours, Mrs T continued to refuse, so a further discussion occurred where all of the information that Mrs T had provided did not reduce the concerns (i.e. she disclosed that she had not been eating but couldn't quantify how long for, whether she had had anything at all to eat, etc.) and so the decision was made that a blood sample would need to be taken against Mrs T's wishes. A team was assembled and briefed as restraining someone to take blood is incredibly dangerous for all involved and so should never be approached lightly in any circumstances. The staff member who had some rapport with Mrs T led the communication and approached Mrs T with the team, explaining that the risk of harm was so high that there was no other choice than to obtain a blood sample from her. It was explained that no one wanted to do this against her will and they understood why she was refusing to consent, but to please reconsider. With the team presence, Mrs T did, very reluctantly, agree to have her bloods taken. It took a significant amount of time to develop a therapeutic relationship with Mrs T as she had ultimately been forced from her home into an unfamiliar environment and had been significantly pressured into having an invasive medical procedure against her will.

Ethically, this is a very difficult situation to face but ultimately, Mrs T could have died if her blood test did not confirm whether she was at risk of refeeding syndrome. The team made a measured decision and had a significant debate about how to proceed in the face of a very difficult situation that no policy could adequately guide you on. Mrs T lacked the capacity to understand the seriousness of the situation due to being unwell and so ultimately, a best interest decision needed to be made. The team had a thorough discussion about what 'the right thing to do' was and every member of the team participated in that discussion. Mrs T did recover well and go home after a few weeks of treatment.

As we can see from this scenario, ethics can be linked to the 'big' situations where it is clear that there is a decision about what is right and what is wrong that needs to be made, but ethics also applies to the 'little' things that happen every day. It may seem like a daunting topic, but all clinical staff are faced with ethical issues every day, so understanding our own ethics and values is key to ensuring we are ethical practitioners.

References

Beauchamp, T.L. and Childress, J.F. (2001) *Principles of biomedical ethics*. USA.

Department of Health (1983). *The Mental Health Act*. Available at: https://www.legislation.gov.uk/ukpga/1983/20 (Accessed: 29 April 2024).

Mandal, J., Ponnambath, D. and Parija, S. (2016) 'Utilitarian and deontological ethics in medicine', *Tropical Parasitology*, 6(1), p. 5. doi: 10.4103/2229-5070.175024.

Milliken, A. and Grace, P. (2015) 'Nurse ethical awareness: Understanding the nature of everyday practice', *Nursing Ethics*, 24(5), pp. 517–524. doi:10.1177/0969733015615172.

Nursing and Midwifery Council (NMC) (2018) *The code: Professional standards of practice and behaviour for nurses, midwives and nursing associates*. London: NMC.

Norvoll, R. and Pedersen, R. (2016) 'Patients' moral views on coercion in mental healthcare', *Nursing Ethics*, 25(6), pp. 796–807. doi:10.1177/0969733016674768.

Roberts M. (2004) 'Psychiatric ethics; a critical introduction for mental health nurses', *Journal of Psychiatric and Mental Health Nursing*, 11(5), pp. 583–588. doi:10.1111/j.1365-2850.2004.00764.x.

Salzmann-Erikson, M. (2018) 'Moral mindfulness: The ethical concerns of healthcare professionals working in a psychiatric intensive care unit', *International Journal of Mental Health Nursing*, 27(6), pp. 1851–1860. doi:10.1111/inm.12494.

Uncu, F. and Güneş, D. (2021) 'The importance of moral sensitivity in nursing education: A comparative study', *Nursing Forum*, 56(3), pp. 635–639. doi:10.1111/nuf.12584.

Williams, D. (2009) 'Forensic nursing and utilitarianism: The quest for being right', *Journal of Forensic Nursing*, 5(1), pp. 49–50. doi:10.1111/j.1939-3938.2009.01031.x.

CHAPTER 18

Working in Teams

In Health and Social Care, we almost always work in teams and even in roles where we may 'lone work', we are still usually connected to a wider team or Multi-Disciplinary Team (MDT). Due to this, team working is an important consideration for any clinician, and we must consider not only our role within a team but also how we can help to improve the team's overall functioning as it has been shown that a well-functioning team is crucial to good patient care (Deacon and Cleary, 2012). Effective teams have improved morale and individuals within the team experience improved job satisfaction (Stevens et al., 2020). Positive team working can also help individuals to cope within difficult and challenging work environments (Deacon and Cleary, 2012), and when we consider how challenging working with mental health in particular can be, the importance of a positive team experience becomes clear. Ultimately, a team can provide a safety net for an individual who may need more support (Cleary et al., 2011). Another core benefit of team working and in particular MDT working is that teams can achieve outcomes that individuals would be unable to achieve alone (Cleary et al., 2011). There can however be numerous challenges to team working including that there can be a blurring of boundaries between roles in an MDT (Horsburgh, Lamdin and Williamson, 2001), and by the nature of team working, there is always an element of conflict.

A frequent critique of healthcare services is poor team working (Deacon and Cleary, 2012), so this highlights the importance of considering not only why good team working is important but also what the key features to team working may be.

Activity

Think back to an experience you have had of working in a team:
- What was your role within the team?
- Do you feel you were a positive influence on the team?
- When did the team work particularly well together? What was the situation and what did the individual members of the team do that you felt helped the team function well?

Thriving in Mental Health Nursing, First Edition. Laura Duncan.
© 2025 John Wiley & Sons Ltd. Published 2025 by John Wiley & Sons Ltd.

- When did the team not work well together? What happened that made you feel like this? What did individuals within the team do or not do that contributed to this?
- How did that team deal with conflict and disagreements? Was this handled in a supportive and respectful manner?

Effective communication is directly related to the success of a team and their goals (Başoğul, 2020) and good communication ultimately needs to start with the leader of any team. Good communication is a key skill of any manager as a team needs to understand plans and decisions effectively to feel well led (Fowler, 2021). The benefits of positive teamwork and collaboration do not just impact the team members themselves, but there is a wider benefit as there are improved patient outcomes, better employee satisfaction, reduced costs and more effective services (Başoğul, 2020).

There are many ways that team working can be improved when it is believed to be sub-optimal. Teamwork training has been evidenced to be very effective in improving team working (Stevens et al., 2020). It has also been shown that an effective way of improving MDT working in particular is for inter-professional learning to begin early on in education settings (Horsburgh, Lamdin and Williamson, 2001) as this builds respect between different professions and helps to understand one's own professional identity and boundaries. This can be particularly important for nurses as the nursing role can at times seem ambiguous as it encompasses such a wide variety of tasks (Terry, 2019). Nurses can at times feel that they are 'in the middle' of other professionals within an MDT (Terry, 2019), and while that could be seen as a negative or cause frustration, it could actually be seen that nurses are the ones to find the balanced perspective and lead on co-ordinating care for the client.

As an individual, it can be challenging to assimilate into a new team (Cleary et al., 2011) and this is something that we can be mindful of when new individuals are joining our team. Those who are effective team workers are collaborative and flexible and have excellent interpersonal skills (Horsburgh, Lamdin and Williamson, 2001). It has also been shown that expressing praise, gratitude and positive team working achievements is an effective way to boost team working (Stevens et al., 2020).

Activity

Positive reinforcement is particularly important to fostering good team working.

Take some time to think about when you have received positive feedback from a member of your team:

- What was the feedback?
- What situation was it in relation to?
- What language did they use to make you feel that this was positive feedback?
- When was the last time you expressed praise or gratitude to a colleague?
- Do you think you express praise and gratitude as frequently as you could/should?
- Do you think this may improve team morale?
- Think of your core team, take some time to reflect on each member of the team and their strengths and positive attitudes. What do they bring to the team? Consider sharing this with them.

Conflict is an important consideration within team working as it can be seen as inevitable, but it is for the leader of the team to ensure conflict is appropriately managed (Başoğul, 2020). Conflict ultimately comes from disagreement (Başoğul, 2020), and if we can recognise that disagreement is a normal and healthy part of any team, it can help us to resolve conflict quickly and effectively. We would never expect to agree with our colleagues and team mates all of the time about every potential situation that could occur and this is why we ultimately should have improved considerations of conflict. We are most likely to experience conflict within our own team and our own clinical environment (Başoğul, 2020), so it is ultimately unavoidable. A key reason that conflict can become more intense or problematic within the team and working environment is that conflict can frequently arise when individuals feel unsupported (Başoğul, 2020). This is ultimately where a disagreement about the best course of action to take can become a much bigger issue within the team. Most people are also very passionate about their role and their clients, and sometimes that passion can lead to more intense feelings about a situation, so we need to reflect on why we may be having strong feelings about a situation when it is occurring.

There are five strategies that can be used to manage conflict: integrating, compromising, dominating, avoiding and obliging (Başoğul, 2020). We will look at a case study that demonstrates each of these individually to help understand each approach better and decide which strategies may be more helpful in producing positive outcomes within the team.

Integrating Case Study

Integrating as an approach occurs when two (or more) parties have a shared goal and have the time and space to think of an appropriate solution.

Chelsea and Jasmine work on a male Psychiatric Intensive Care Unit (PICU) and are the two nurses on shift. They have just been informed by their manager that the other PICU in the trust has been having issues and needs to swap a service user because they have two individuals who cannot be on the same ward any longer. The ward manager has asked Chelsea and Jasmine to decide who they should transfer to make space for their new admission.

Chelsea and Jasmine sit in the office to discuss and identify that there are several things that they need to consider, and they write down the questions they feel they need to answer:

- Should we agree to the transfer?
- Do we know everything we should about the person being transferred?
- Should we send the person who is most settled right now and if so, who is that?
- Who would want to be transferred?
- Should we try and resolve any conflicts between clients on our own ward?
- Do we know if this is going to be for a specific amount of time?
- What paperwork do we need to do?
- Is there anyone else we should inform in the decision?

They spend time discussing each point and decide that they should transfer Ben. Ben has been doing really well on the ward and will be ready for discharge soon, but he has been having some issues with another client on the ward who has been rude to him repeatedly. Due to this, Chelsea and Jasmine think that Ben will be very happy to move to another ward. They approach their manager to confirm their thoughts and decision; they then discuss with Ben who is very happy to be moving to another ward. Chelsea and Jasmine decide that Chelsea will manage their paperwork and planning for the transfer of Ben and Jasmine will be in charge of the client being admitted to their ward. Jasmine calls the other PICU, requests some additional information and confirms the plan for transfer. The transfers go smoothly, and Chelsea and Jasmine reflect later that they're glad they approached the situation in the manner that they did.

As you can see in that scenario, having time to plan and discuss was crucial for an 'integrating' approach. Chelsea and Jasmine worked together as a team, and they listened to each other's perspectives and divided the tasks, so they both felt supported and motivated in the scenario. They took the time to reflect and recognise that they'd done a good job and had worked together well, which reinforced the good team working further.

Compromising Case Study

Compromising is probably one of the most common approaches to conflict and the one we are likely most familiar with. Compromise is about finding a solution that may not be what any party actually wants to happen, but there is some sense of balance and even if reluctant, agreement.

Mike is the band six of an acute ward and is in charge of the rota. There are nine Band 5's on the ward team currently, and all of them have requested to have Christmas and New Year off. Mike has already sent a team message saying that it will not be possible for everyone to get the time they have requested off, and for the sake of fairness, no one will be off on both Christmas and New Year. The team is unhappy but understands the situation.

Of the nine nurses, eight have said that they would have Christmas off rather than New Years, which has not made the situation much easier for Mike. The nurse who has said she doesn't mind working on Christmas if she can have New Years off is rostered for Christmas Eve and Christmas Day on a long day. She will be off for New Year's Eve and New Year's Day. Of the other nurses, Mike decides that he will use short shifts to balance it out, so each of the nurses is on either an early or a late shift on Christmas Eve, Christmas Day and Boxing Day. The nurses reluctantly agree that this is the fairest solution but ask if they can swap shifts amongst themselves as long as each shift remains covered, and Mike agrees to this.

As you can see in this scenario (which I imagine happens every year on every ward!), it is a situation that cannot have everyone happy and satisfied with the outcome. None of the nurses were going to be happy with working over Christmas, but they all compromised to ensure the needs of the service were met and it was fair amongst them all. If Mike had have said that his considerations would have been down to who had children, who asked first, etc., then that could lead to issues within the team. If the ward operates a 'first come, first served' plan for festive leave, anyone who joins the team later in the year is immediately disadvantaged.

With a compromised solution, ultimately no one is 100% happy with the outcome, but as long as the reasonings and justifications are communicated, then people do tend to be understanding.

Dominating Case Study

Dominating as an approach can be quite difficult to manage in an appropriate way, and it can feel very challenging if you are the one on the receiving end. It can be appropriate though when someone who may have more knowledge, expertise or responsibility in a scenario would have to justify their decision-making or knows that other suggestions are inappropriate. If the scenario needs a fast solution and there is no time to discuss, then a dominating approach may be needed.

Sadiq is a male in his late 20s who has been admitted to an inpatient ward for 3 weeks with no known physical health issues. Sadiq is in the corridor and collapses. A Health Care Assistant (HCA), Jenny, witnesses Sadiq's collapse and activates their alarm. The team quickly responds, and Natasha as the nurse in charge of the shift takes charge of the situation. Natasha asks Jenny to call 2222, seek assistance and ask for an ambulance to be called. Jenny says they don't think an ambulance is necessary, and he probably just needs water or something. Natasha tells Jenny that she is the nurse in charge and an ambulance needs to be called immediately. Jenny reluctantly goes to make the call and Natasha requests another member of the team bring the crash trolley so observations can be done. The ambulance arrives, and Sadiq is taken to The Emergency Department.

Natasha leads the de-brief with the team once Sadiq has been safely escorted from the ward. Jenny says that she is very upset with the way Natasha spoke to her and feels Natasha should have listened to her perspective. Natasha politely advises Jenny that this was a medical emergency, and as the nurse in charge of the shift, it was her decision to make and that it was her responsibility. Natasha apologises for upsetting Jenny and says that she didn't mean to hurt her feelings, but she had to take charge of the situation and that her decision was correct. Natasha later has a 1:1 discussion with Jenny to reflect on the scenario and what to do during medical emergencies. Jenny reluctantly agrees that she understands an ambulance was needed in the scenario and that it was Natasha's decision to make.

As you can see, dominating can lead to bad feeling within the team; in the scenario of a medical emergency, most could understand the need to use a dominating approach. If there was a scenario where there wasn't such an urgent situation, it can feel like 'pulling rank' if not explained appropriately.

Avoiding Case Study

Avoiding conflict is sometimes the natural response from many people, but it generally doesn't feel as though it is an actual 'strategy' to deal with conflict; however, it can be.

Sasha is a care co-ordinator for Bobby and is discussing his case with the team. Sasha reports that she went to visit Bobby and he swore at her and told her to go away, refusing to accept his depot at the same time. Sasha thinks Bobby needs admitting to an inpatient ward as in her opinion, he is clearly deteriorating and cannot be managed safely in the community. Annabelle has known Bobby for a long time and has worked with him on and off for several years. Annabelle feels that even when unwell, Bobby would never swear at anyone unless he felt they had been rude to him first, so Annabelle says that to Sasha. Sasha takes offence to this and believes Annabelle is saying that she has been unprofessional. Annabelle and Sasha both get upset. Annabelle abruptly walks away and leaves the room. Sasha is very angry and states to other members of the team that she can't believe Annabelle just walked away from her.

Later that day, Annabelle approaches Sasha and says that she apologises for walking away, but she felt it was a better choice than continuing the argument when she was feeling very emotional as she did not want to make the situation worse. Sasha is clearly still very upset and explains to Annabelle that she was looking for her team to support her and give her advice about the situation with Bobby as she too was very surprised that he was rude to her but felt that Annabelle was insinuating she had done something to deserve it. Annabelle advises that she understands that that was how it came across and that she didn't mean that, but she was just very surprised at Bobby's behaviour and didn't take a step back to think about it before speaking. She asks Sasha if there anything she can do to help with the situation with Bobby and suggests maybe they could do a joint visit to see how he is and make a decision as to whether he would benefit from an inpatient admission. Sasha agrees to this plan and the two arrange to see Bobby together the next day.

In this scenario, emotions became intense and that is when avoiding becomes the most appropriate option. If we feel ourselves becoming emotional, then taking some time to calm down and reflect on why it was so emotionally triggering can help us move forward more constructively. If Annabelle had not removed herself from the situation, it could have continued escalating and could have permanently damaged Annabelle and Sasha's working relationship.

Obliging Case Study

Obliging can be an interesting approach to conflict management and is usually seen when the situation is ultimately of little consequence to the person who is obliging. It can be a helpful approach in terms of 'picking your battles' or finding a very quick solution.

Effie is the nurse in charge and completing the allocations for the shift. The ward is short staffed and two service users have appointments in the general hospital at different points of the day. Effie asks Janice to come to the office and explains she is having difficulties with making the allocations seem fair for everyone. Effie explains that as there is ward round happening, she needs to keep herself and the other nurse, Bola, on the ward, leaving Janice and John as the HCAs on shift. As John is the only male on shift, Effie wouldn't want him to leave the ward, and as the two service users who need escorting to appointments are female, it feels that Janice is the best choice. Effie apologises and states that she knows doing both escorts will be busy and stressful but doesn't feel there is any other solution. Janice says that she understands and can't see a better solution either, so will do both escorts. Effie thanks her for being so understanding and a team player. Effie says that Janice can have first pick of duties next time they are on shift together as a thank you for being so accommodating.

In this scenario, Janice would have been fully justified in expressing her discontent at the situation or even refusing to oblige at all. Effie handled the situation well by explaining the issue she was facing and what her considerations were so that Janice felt that she had been consulted about the matter and part of the decision-making process, even if she did oblige Effie in the end. By obliging in this situation, Janice has shown that she is a good team player and this will help her working relationship with Effie in particular. This will also mean that in situations of conflict in future, if Janice does express a strong opinion or feeling about a matter, Effie is more likely to oblige to her or compromise as she knows that Janice will oblige when appropriate.

In summary, team working is a core consideration to all of our roles within health and social care as there are very few roles where you would not be working within a team. As we have seen, good team working leads to improved patient care and outcomes (Stevens et al., 2020) which is ultimately what we all should be striving for. Good quality care can only be provided when there is a team that manages conflict effectively (Başoğul, 2020) and although avoiding can be a valid strategy to manage conflict, pretending it does not/will not happen is not a valid strategy. To develop a strong team that works well together, we need to consider our own individual role within the team and think about whether we are a positive influence. Are we being the team member that we would want others to be? Positive reinforcement to our team mates is incredibly important as it improves morale but also makes sure individuals feel acknowledged and valued. Teamwork can also help with positive role modelling (Cleary et al., 2011) as we can learn from others who are strong team players as well as role model to those whose team working could be improved. A strong, supportive and well-functioning team ultimately starts with a leader who understands the importance of communicating effectively and supporting their team to grow and develop. As seen in the case studies above, all of the scenarios had positive outcomes when there was good communication demonstrated. We cannot avoid conflict or disagreement; particularly, when people are passionate about their roles, it can become emotive and heated, but a strong leader who understands how to manage conflict effectively can channel that passion into positive outcomes.

References

Başoğul, C. (2020) 'Conflict management and teamwork in workplace from the perspective of Nurses', *Perspectives in Psychiatric Care*, 57(2), pp. 610–619. doi:10.1111/ppc.12584.

Cleary, M. et al. (2011) 'Valuing teamwork: Insights from newly-registered nurses working in specialist mental health services', *International Journal of Mental Health Nursing*, 20(6), pp. 454–459. doi:10.1111/j.1447-0349.2011.00752.x.

Deacon, M. and Cleary, M. (2012) 'The reality of teamwork in an acute mental health ward', *Perspectives in Psychiatric Care*, 49(1), pp. 50–57. doi:10.1111/j.1744-6163.2012.00340.x.

Fowler, J. (2021) 'Team working part 4: Managing a team', *British Journal of Nursing*, 30(16), pp. 988–988. doi:10.12968/bjon.2021.30.16.988.

Horsburgh, M., Lamdin, R. and Williamson, E. (2001) 'Multiprofessional learning: The attitudes of medical, nursing and pharmacy students to shared learning', *Medical Education*, 35(9), pp. 876–883. doi:10.1046/j.1365-2923.2001.00959.x.

Stevens, M. et al. (2020) 'Becoming a high-performing team', *Nursing Management*, 51(9), pp. 14–18. doi:10.1097/01.numa.0000694900.00441.7b.

Terry, J. (2019) '"In the middle": A qualitative study of talk about mental health nursing roles and work', *International Journal of Mental Health Nursing*, 29(3), pp. 414–426. doi:10.1111/inm.12676.

CHAPTER 19

Leadership

Leadership is crucial within all aspects of health and social care, but we frequently forget that not all managers are leaders, and not all leaders are managers. We can lead from any level of an organisation, and good leadership skills can have significant benefit to not only the team but also the clients. Nurses are expected to be clinical leaders, and good clinical leadership skills are linked to improved outcomes for clients and better retention of staff (Ennis, Happell and Reid-Searl, 2014). One of the most important aspects of what we consider to be 'good leadership' is that it creates environments where staff can practice confidently, without fear and anxiety (Foye, 2019). This is because with effective and compassionate leadership, the team does not fear a 'blame culture' and feels comfortable and confident in raising their concerns or issues without feeling as though they will be criticised or punished. A team that feels they can express their thoughts and feelings and admit any mistakes or errors that may occur is going to be a stronger and more resilient team. The team that fears their manager is more likely to hide any mistakes or errors rather than being honest and transparent which is the antithesis of the NMC code (2018) and is likely to lead to poor practice and lower standards of care.

All nurses having positive leadership skills is important due to the 24/7 nature of nursing care in particular. Nurses are the professionals most likely to face unexpected or unplanned scenarios during their working hours (Ennis, Happell and Reid-Searl, 2014). It can be daunting as an early-career nurse to be 'Nurse in Charge', but positive role modelling and confidence in your own leadership skills can make this significantly less challenging when it occurs.

Positive and compassionate leadership is particularly important in nursing as research has shown that the mental health of nurses has significantly declined since the pandemic and rates of stress, anxiety and depression are higher amongst nurses than in the general population pre-pandemic (Stelnicki and Carleton, 2021). Poor mental health can lead to burnout, and burnout is a significant concern for organisational leaders as it is believed to lead to diminished quality and safety of care (Lown, Shin and Jones, 2019). Good quality leadership is also crucial for the recruitment and retention of staff (Ennis, Happell and Reid-Searl, 2015) as people will leave poor

Thriving in Mental Health Nursing, First Edition. Laura Duncan.
© 2025 John Wiley & Sons Ltd. Published 2025 by John Wiley & Sons Ltd.

leaders that they don't feel safe and confident working with. We are currently in the midst of a workforce crisis where early- and mid-career nurses are leaving the profession in significant numbers, which highlights the importance of these groups in particular needing to feel valued and that they are a priority for clinical and senior leaders (Berry, 2023). Leaders must advocate for and action change to protect the nursing workforce (Stelnicki and Carleton, 2021). One way to ensure early- and mid-career nurses feel valued and supported is ensuring that all nurses and leaders support their education and development and this should be seen as a key role for all nurses (Ennis, Happell and Reid-Searl, 2015). Leadership can make a significant difference not only to staff but also to clients involved with mental health care services (Mildon et al., 2017), so its importance and relevance to every professional's practice should never be underestimated.

Having considered why leadership is important, we will now look at different types of leadership and how they can look in practice. There have been countless authors who have contributed to the discussion around leadership styles since Kurt Lewin in 1939 created the first three styles of leadership. Below is a discussion of what are commonly accepted as the key leadership styles and their strengths and weaknesses from the International Institute for Management Development (IMD, 2023):

- Transformational leadership – This leadership style embraces change, and these leaders are seen as inspiring by their teams. They focus strongly on the future, change and people. While change is always important, this style of leadership can miss the good practice that may already exist in their quest to always be moving forward and improving services.
- Delegative leaders – They are also sometimes referred to as 'Laissez-Faire', and it is generally considered a 'hands-off' style. These leaders don't micromanage, and this can be a very positive approach for a team that is experienced, competent and diligent. If there are issues that need to be addressed, this style can struggle to manage complex situations and be 'hands-on' when needed.
- Authoritative leaders – They see themselves as mentors, and they focus on motivating and inspiring others. This can be a strong leadership style when working with early-career teams but for more experienced staff, it can lead to micromanaging and frustration as authoritative leaders don't tend to recognise the strengths and expertise of others easily.
- Transactional leadership – This style focuses on reward and punishment. This can be effective in environments like sales where reaching a certain target may lead to a financial bonus as the incentive but is a challenging approach in healthcare as there are limited rewards that could be offered without becoming unethical. Simply punishing by criticism or negative feedback isn't 'transactional', it is just negative! The basis of this leadership style is that there is the opportunity for reward.
- Participative leadership – It is also known as 'democratic leadership', and in this style, leaders listen to the team and actively involve others in the decision making process. This leadership style creates good collaboration and makes team members feel valued and respected, but the participative leader must have excellent communication skills to adopt this leadership style effectively.

- Servant leadership – This style puts the needs of others first and focusses on building strong relationships to help people reach their full potential. Problem solving and creativity can flourish with this leadership style, and it is believed to build loyalty within the team as all members of the team feel appreciated and listened to. A servant leader can struggle when there are issues within the team that require direct management or performance management however.

If you ask most people which leadership style they are or would like to demonstrate, they will say 'Transformational', which sounds very positive and motivating. However, we should not see leadership styles as a binary choice, where we are one and that is all we are. There will be times when 'Transformational' is the absolute best approach, you are leading a new team in a brand new service and they need you to be change-focussed and inspiring. Five years later, however, the service is running well, feedback is excellent, clients feel well supported and the team is experienced, established and competent. Transformational isn't quite so needed now; in this scenario, you may need to be more 'Delegative', 'Participative' or 'Servant' in your leadership style. You may need to adapt your leadership style for different members of the team; the newly qualified nurse on their first day with the team will need a different approach and level of support to the nurse who has been in their role and has been excellent at their job for the last 10 years. The key point is that one style does not fit all scenarios and people; we need to understand the different approaches and make a considered decision as to which approach is best for the person, team and scenario at hand. Making an active decision to be 'Delegative' is very different to not leading or participating, and it has its time and place where it is an appropriate and valid choice to make. The very best leaders will be able to recognise who needs which approach from them and when to change their approach to match the needs of their team and service.

Although there are lots of different approaches to leadership style, one thing it should always be is compassionate. Creating a compassionate and supportive culture is crucial for people to thrive (Trueland, 2022) in their professional and personal lives. In mental health services, staff are frequently exposed to challenging situations, trauma and unfortunately, violence or abuse in their roles which is why we must focus on compassionate leadership. Leaders need to provide space to talk about the emotionally challenging aspects of the role including when teams have experienced suicide or self-harm (Foye, 2019) as although these may occur or be discussed frequently in some clinical environments, it can always be distressing or upsetting to be exposed or witness to. As well as providing appropriate space to discuss challenging situations and leading good quality de-briefs, effective leaders are able to demonstrate a calm and confident approach to clinical situations which has a positive influence on colleagues and team members (Ennis, Happell and Reid-Searl, 2014). Leading by example is a core tenant in compassionate leadership (Trueland, 2022) as is role modelling. Role modelling is an important factor in the professional development of ourselves and others as we will ensure our behaviour is that which we would like to see and be emulated by others, knowing that we are being observed and that our actions are likely to be mirrored (Ennis, Happell and Reid-Searl, 2015) which means that if we demonstrate compassionate leadership to others, we are more likely to see compassionate leadership from others. Compassionate leaders are supportive of their teams and prioritise inclusivity (Trueland, 2022) as feeling able to be ourselves is crucial in being comfortable with our leaders and teams. Professionalism, honesty, being approachable and wanting to share their knowledge and experience are all traits identified as key features of a good clinical leader (Ennis, Happell and Reid-Searl, 2015), but these traits also align with compassionate leadership.

There are four key behaviours associated with compassionate leadership (Trueland, 2022):

- Attending – This means to be present to actively listen and focus on the person/people with whom you are interacting.
- Understanding – This involves taking time to explore and consider the needs of those around you, not only the team but also the clients and services that may also be impacted by your decisions as a leader. This involves ensuring you have all the relevant information to make a decision or take action.
- Empathising – You need to be able to recognise the feelings and emotions of your team, and you should be able to consider the emotional impact of any actions or decisions and accept that people will and do have feelings
- Helping – This involves taking actions that are thoughtful and are intended to help the team perform and function more healthily.

Thinking of the thoughts and feelings of others is crucial in mental health services due to the nature of the work we do, but frequently we forget this when we become leaders and managers. As discussed by Trueland (2022), being empathetic is a core factor in compassionate leadership. Another key consideration as leaders should be to 'lift as you climb'. Supporting and mentoring junior colleagues is a key feature of leadership roles, and we should want our colleagues to thrive and succeed. Others succeeding does not threaten our own success; rather, it actually strengthens our bonds and reputation, so when you see an opportunity to help someone else develop, take it.

Case Studies

The following case studies are intended to demonstrate what good and effective leadership looks like and feels like to those around them. The first example is from when I was newly qualified in my first Band 5 role; I think it was actually my first week, so I really was brand new. The second example is from several years later working in a very different environment in many different ways. The third and final example was from my time as a support worker, before undertaking my nurse training.

When I think about 'Compassionate Leadership', I have a very clear example in my mind of the person who embodies this approach in everything they did. My modern matron when I was first qualified is a prime example, and she was one of the kindest, most thoughtful and supportive people I have ever come across. One of the many examples I could give of her demonstrating compassionate leadership was I think one of our earliest one-to-one meetings when I had first started working for her. She asked me generally how I was feeling being brand new to the service, etc., and

I remember vividly talking about how nervous and panicked I was, that I didn't feel ready. The feelings that most new Band 5's have in their first weeks in new roles; the imposter syndrome was strong. She was so reassuring and calmed me down; now I think back, she must have worked with hundreds of brand new nurses in her career, so my little panic was nothing new to her.

One of the very concrete things I remember was telling her that I didn't feel confident with wound care at all. The ward that I was working on at that time was a triage assessment unit, so all admissions in the borough would go through that ward. What that meant was that everyone there was in crisis and acutely unwell, and unfortunately, a lot of people had self-harmed before being admitted or would try to hurt themselves whilst on the ward, meaning that there actually was a significant need for good wound care skills. She reassured me in the way that I now emulate on a very regular basis that no one feels confident when they first qualify and you can never feel completely confident in every aspect of nursing. She also told me that when someone needed wound care the next time, she would work with me to help build my skills and confidence. She was a modern matron who was actually in charge of several high intensity, challenging and demanding services, but she made time to have that conversation and then actually help me with the issue I was worrying about. A day or so later, there was a gentleman admitted and he had cut himself all over his arms and torso; in total, there must have been over 300 individual lacerations. Each individual laceration needed cleaning, reviewing and dressing if necessary. Many of them were scratches that didn't require further intervention, but in total, we were in the treatment room with him for a couple of hours. She let me lead, and whilst I was cleaning and assessing the wounds, I was talking to the gentleman who really opened up about what it meant to him, why he would cut himself and how distressing he found hearing voices; by the end of the session, we had developed a really positive therapeutic relationship. We had talked at length about his experiences and what he would like to happen next, etc., which could then inform his care and care plan moving forward.

My matron didn't intervene at any point; she watched and participated in the discussion, and if I wasn't sure about a specific cut, whether it needed a dressing or not, for example, she would reflect it back to me and ask what I thought. After we had finished, I asked her for feedback and she was very positive. She told me I'd done a really good job and had no reason to doubt my skills. In reality, as there were so many wounds, I probably did make some mistakes or not do it perfectly (obviously nothing significant or she would have intervened and corrected me), but in that moment, she knew it was more important for me to build confidence than specific skills. If I were in her position now, I would be most keen to see a nurse who was kind, gentle and supportive of the client who was in a very emotional and vulnerable position.

I walked away from that afternoon feeling much more positive and confident, which is obviously a great outcome, but most importantly, I never worried about asking her for help. I knew, because she had demonstrated this very clearly, that if I wasn't sure or wasn't confident, she would help me. I never worried about telling her if I had made a mistake or an error because I trusted her as a leader to respond appropriately and proportionately. She also knew that because of this, she could trust me as a junior staff member to say if I wasn't sure about something and that I would escalate anything necessary. One aspect of leadership that isn't really addressed in the literature is that notion of trust; if you are leading me, I need to trust that you are competent and able to do that, but as a leader, you also need to trust your team to be able to do their jobs well and to escalate anything necessary as and when it happens. That matron is still one of my favourite people I've ever worked with and I frequently find myself asking 'what would she do in this situation?'. She is the ultimate role model for me, and I genuinely believe I've been a much better nurse throughout my career for having such a compassionate leader at the very start of it.

142 Chapter 19 Leadership

The next case study isn't so immediately clear in terms of 'this is great leadership' as it was a very complex and nuanced situation. I was working for an organisation that really did prioritise their staff's development and support, which was excellent. It was a slightly unusual set up in terms of I didn't actually work alongside anyone else from my organisation but instead worked alongside clinicians from a different organisation. This was challenging for a couple of reasons, but slowly over time, it became intolerable. The clinician I had to work most closely with was awful to me and treated me appallingly. Her team seemed to always back her up even when they knew that she had lied or created a situation deliberately. I honestly cannot tell you her motivation or why she disliked me so intensely, but I begged to be moved location. I would cry on my way home (which was a 2-hour and three-train commute!) most days, and although I loved my role, I couldn't continue to work with her.

I initially had one manager who had basically been through the same torment as I had with this particular individual which basically meant they were not in a place where they could support me effectively because they were already dealing with their own issues with this team. I asked her to move me locations or to help every time I saw her after my first month and was given lots of kind and supportive words, but ultimately I needed action to be taken. I had been keeping a log of every incident diligently, and she was aware of this. That manager then left the organisation, and I got a new manager. They asked if there were any issues they needed to be aware of, and I honestly remember laughing because I thought she was joking. When she didn't know why I was laughing, it became clear that my previous manager had not shared my issues or concerns with anyone else in the management team. I sent my new manager the log I had been keeping, and when I spoke to her the next day, she said she was so upset and angry that all of this had happened and nothing had been done.

Having now been in that situation, and utterly miserable, for 11 months, I was beyond thrilled that my new manager was taking the issue seriously and wanted to help me. She went to her manager for support, and they arranged a meeting with the other team's senior leadership. I had had many a conversation with these individuals; they were fully aware of the issues and problems that I was having, but in that meeting, they said they knew nothing of the issues and had no idea what it was about.

My manager and her manager took me for a coffee, and I remember them being utterly bewildered at what had happened; they told me they would go back to the drawing board and come up with a new plan, just bear with them. I knew in that moment that it was all going to get immediately worse. I hate being right sometimes. I returned to my office and was immediately being screamed at. I went home that night, and the minute I left, I just sobbed. I cried all night and was in an awful state in the morning, but I knew I couldn't continue. I had left things in the office, so I went and sent an email saying that I simply could not continue like this and I would go and work at another location, go to head office or they could fire me, but I would not be staying there. I received almost an immediate response from senior management and went to head office to meet with them.

They apologised that they hadn't known just how bad the whole situation was and should have realised that after their meeting, it would have worsened, so they should have told me to leave then. We agreed I would finish my log of incidents and send it to them and then go to work in another location as of the next day.

The new location was much better; the team were great, and there were none of those kind of issues. The other organisation 'investigated', did not pursue any action with any of the individuals involved and offered me mediation, which believe it or not, I refused. About a week into working at the new location, totally unrelated to anything that had previously happened, I was the subject of gang threats (actually nothing to do with me, my name just got attached!) which meant I was advised by the police to take different routes home, be vigilant, etc. The gang members were persistently attending my work location, trying to find me, and it was genuinely very frightening.

I had attended a supervision on the Friday of this week and was very emotional because it had been a very tough week. On the Monday morning, when I went to the new location, one of my managers was there and told me to go home and take the rest of the week off. I told her I was fine, I could work, it was busy, etc., but she insisted and I did. I didn't really realise it until a few days later, but I very much did need to take a break.

There are lots of issues and errors in this example of where things were not handled as well as they could have been, but we actually don't learn how to be good leaders focussing on negative examples. Instead, we will draw out the positives, of which there were many. Manager number 2 immediately recognised the seriousness of the situation; they understood and wanted to help; they involved the senior manager straight away, and action was taken. When that action didn't have the desired outcome and led to the worsening of the situation for me, they apologised. It wasn't their fault that this whole situation had happened, but they knew they should have removed me from that location that day. Apologising very genuinely made me feel more supported; I felt like they actually cared about how I felt and my wellbeing. They then did move me, which was probably quite challenging in terms of logistics and needs of the service, but my wellbeing was prioritised in that scenario. That is an example of excellent leadership. After I had unrelated issues at the new location (it was just bad luck!) and was very emotional during my clinical supervision, it became clear to my whole management team that I was not coping well, so they took action and told me to take the next week off.

From a leader and manager perspective, this is one of the most challenging types of situations you could face. Two individuals are not getting along in quite an extreme way; although there is a history of and evidence of their poor conduct, you cannot take any action because they are not within your organisation. You instead have to raise and escalate what you can, hoping the other organisation takes appropriate steps (which they did not) and attempt to support your staff member when you can't resolve the issue they are facing. Now I reflect on it from the manager and leadership perspective; it must have been so difficult to know what to do. Ultimately, they recognised that I was suffering in this situation and they tried to support me as best as they could.

Obviously, that was a very difficult period for me in my career, but had I not have taken that week off, had they not have moved me to a new location, I would have ended up quitting and moving on to a new role elsewhere. I can't say the next three years in that role were all smooth sailing, but I stayed, I did my job and I enjoyed it. If my managers hadn't have supported me, tried to take action and made me feel valued, that wouldn't have been the situation.

The third case study is from when I was new to the field of mental health and had started a role as a support worker on a Psychiatric Intensive Care Unit (PICU). I had no formal background or training in mental health, but I had volunteered for several years with a charity that supported individuals with mental health issues. I had no idea what to expect from that role, but I absolutely loved it. The team was amazing and the leadership was outstanding. I didn't fully appreciate it at the time, but I was so supported and nurtured while I worked with that team that I genuinely wouldn't be where I am now without them, so if you're reading, thank you!

I was asked if I would like to attend a conference with some other members of the team, including the ward manager, which I was thrilled about as I'd never been to a conference before, so it was all very exciting. We went to the conference, and in one of the talks, I learned about a quality improvement project that other PICUs had adopted with great success. I was really inspired by it and thought it would work on our unit well. I explained it to my ward manager later, and he told me he agreed; it sounded great, but he wanted me to get more details and liaise with the person who had been presenting to arrange a visit to their PICU who had already done this project. I remember immediately being terrified of having to approach the presenter. I did it though, and he was happy for our team to come and visit. I found out more and presented the details to my manager; he agreed it sounded really positive.

The core focus of this project was to work in sub-teams, and it needed co-ordination to make it run smoothly; the ward manager told me to go ahead and co-ordinate it and make it happen. Of course, the whole team was involved, and we had great success with it, but it was my proposal, I led on it and I saw it to completion.

Most managers would not give that level of responsibility to someone so junior and new to the field, my manager did. He saw I was passionate and enthusiastic and let me run with it. He taught me an incredible lesson in that moment that my job title, age, gender, experience, etc., didn't define me. I was just as capable as others to complete certain tasks, and my energy and enthusiasm frequently meant that I could find improvements that would be positive for everyone. He recognised that me progressing and succeeding at something in no way threatened him; in fact, it actually would reflect well on him that even his most junior and inexperienced staff were making positive change. This is the epitome of 'lift as you climb'. He had legitimate authority that meant he was in control of whether this project happened and who led on it, he could have taken the project for himself, so he could claim credit, he could have given it to someone else who was more senior or experienced than me, but instead, he knew this was a development opportunity for me. He recognised that this would teach me to lead, to delegate and to complete a complex and long-term task. He knew this would help me in my future career, and instead of being threatened by that, he actively encouraged me and supported me to complete it.

As we have considered the different styles of leadership, what it is and is not and considered some examples in real life of leadership, now we will focus on how to develop our own leadership skills. As discussed earlier, we can be leaders at any level of an organisation; you do not need to have formal management responsibilities to be a leader.

Activity

Think of the last time you led something. It could have been a specific task, group work, a shift, anything that you may have been involved in where you feel you took the lead.

- Take some time to consider:
    - What was the goal in that situation?
    - Did you achieve the goal?
    - What could have been improved upon?
    - What leadership style do you think you adopted?
    - Do you think that was the best style for the situation?
    - Was there a style that would have been particularly bad for that situation? What do you think would have been the outcome if you had used that style?
    - How did the people you were leading respond to you?
    - What do you think they would say about your leadership style?

Completing that activity will hopefully have identified some of your strengths as a leader already but you also should have considered how you are perceived by others when leading. As we have established, leadership involves other people and success as a leader is very much in the eye of those being led.

- Take some time to consider who has been the most compassionate leader you have worked with and make notes about:
  - Who were they?
  - When did they lead you?
  - Were they a manager as well as a leader?
  - What made their leadership feel compassionate?
  - What actions did they take to make you feel supported?
  - How would they handle a challenging situation?
  - How would they support a team member who was upset?
  - How would they handle a complaint about a team member?
  - How would they manage someone who was not performing their role adequately?

You may not have witnessed the compassionate leader you were thinking of do all of these things, but you are likely to have a good idea of how they would approach different scenarios and you can use your thoughts on this to role model your own compassionate leadership skills.

As mental health nurses, we demonstrate empathy, compassion and active listening skills every day, but we frequently forget that these skills are the same needed to be a good leader. We must remember that our teams are made up of humans, who may have significant challenges happening in their personal lives that could impact their professional performance. We know from our own experiences that having a supportive manager can make an incredible difference. We can recognise those people who helped us develop our knowledge and skills, who shared theirs and built our confidence. By reflecting on the good leaders we have experienced, we can role model from them and develop our skills further. Acknowledging the strengths and skills for others will never diminish our own, so the same way we can look up to others for guidance, support and leadership and we can share our own with junior colleagues to 'lift as you climb'.

References

Berry, L. (2023) 'Compassionate mental healthcare relies on a valued workforce' *Mental Health Practice*, 26(3), pp. 5–5. doi:10.7748/mhp.26.3.5.s1.

Ennis, G., Happell, B. and Reid-Searl, K. (2014) 'Clinical leadership in mental health nursing: The importance of a calm and confident approach', *Perspectives in Psychiatric Care*, 51(1), pp. 57–62. doi:10.1111/ppc.12070.

Ennis, G., Happell, B. and Reid-Searl, K. (2015) 'Enabling professional development in mental health nursing: The role of clinical leadership', *Journal of Psychiatric and Mental Health Nursing*, 22(8), pp. 616–622. doi:10.1111/jpm.12221.

Foye, U. (2019) 'Nursing leaders should try to champion holistic care', *Nursing Management*, 26(6), pp. 13–13. doi:10.7748/nm.26.6.13.s9.

IMD (2023) *The 6 most common leadership styles & how to find yours, IMD business school for management and leadership courses*. International Institute for Management Development. Available at: https://www.imd.org/reflections/leadership-styles/ (Accessed: 4 December 2023).

Lown, B. A., Shin, A. and Jones, R. N. (2019) 'Can organizational leaders sustain compassionate, patient-centered care and mitigate burnout?', *Journal of Healthcare Management*, 64(6), pp. 398–412. doi:10.1097/jhm-d-18-00023.

Mildon, B., Cleverley, K., Strudwick, G., Srivastava, R. and Velji, K. (2017) 'Nursing leadership: Making a difference in mental health', *Canadian Journal of Nursing Leadership*, 30(3), pp. 8–22. doi:10.12927/cjnl.2018.25388.

Nursing and Midwifery Council (NMC) (2018) *The code: Professional standards of practice and behaviour for nurses, midwives and nursing associates*. London: NMC.

Stelnicki, A. and Carleton, R. (2021) 'Nursing leadership has an important role in the management of Nurses' mental health', *Canadian Journal of Nursing Leadership*, 34(2), pp. 12–15. doi:10.12927/cjnl.2021.26537.

Trueland, J. (2022) 'Making compassionate leadership a reality', *Mental Health Practice*, 25(6), pp. 8–9. doi:10.7748/mhp.25.6.8.s4.

CHAPTER 20

Supervision Skills

Clinical supervision has been a standard part of nursing practice since the early 1990s (Bowles and Young, 1999), but what it actually means and how it occurs are still somewhat changeable or misunderstood. Access to good clinical supervision is inconsistent across health and social care services (Jones, 2023), and there are issues regarding the level of training that clinical supervisors receive, if any (Turner and Hill, 2011). The difference between clinical supervision and managerial supervision in nursing is inconsistent, and many nurses see clinical supervision as the same thing as line management supervision which focuses on performance (Jones, 2023); however, the benefits of supervision are multifaceted and include improving care quality by gaining greater understanding and the sharing of knowledge, skills and information (Tuck, 2017). Clinical supervision is well recognised as a tool to support nurses to build and reflect on their practice (Jones, 2023). Clinical supervision however cannot make up for poor management or poor clinical environments (White and Winstanley, 2021), so if issues are identified within clinical supervision, the supervisee should be supported to raise and escalate these to the appropriate person.

There are significant differences between managerial and clinical supervisions even though there may be overlap or they may be performed by the same individual. A line management supervision will normally be undertaken by your direct superior, the frequency of which will be determined by the organisation and there will normally be a set agenda that will focus on performance of clinical duties and other measurable factors such as completion of mandatory training. Clinical supervision however should be undertaken by a professional of your choosing and will be more reflective in nature (Jones, 2023). The majority of nurses will generally look outside of their own clinical area and will usually go to someone senior to them, but this is not always the case (Bowles and Young, 1999). There can be many benefits to choosing a clinical supervisor outside of your clinical area, but the key factor in choosing a clinical supervisor should be that it is someone that you are comfortable with, whose opinion you respect and someone that you trust and feel can be a role model to you. The key skills

Thriving in Mental Health Nursing, First Edition. Laura Duncan.
© 2025 John Wiley & Sons Ltd. Published 2025 by John Wiley & Sons Ltd.

identified for clinical supervisors to possess are excellent listening and communication skills as they may need to support their supervisee during times of stress or distress (Jones, 2023). Studies also suggest that those who have been clinical supervisors for longer have improved supervision outcomes (Bowles and Young, 1999). These are all important considerations when choosing your own clinical supervisor.

Clinical supervision is generally more 'ad hoc' and less structured in terms of time than managerial supervision and has a stronger focus on wellbeing. Many nurses prefer more informal methods of supervision such as ad hoc and talking to a colleague for peer support (Jones, 2023). Group or team clinical supervision has been shown to have many benefits and is linked to improved self-awareness and empathy towards peers as well as assisting in developing reflective skills (Sheppard, Stacey and Aubeeluck, 2018); however, in most clinical areas, team supervision isn't formalised and usually only occurs spontaneously or sporadically (Tuck, 2017). The most common example of this is during a de-brief following a significant or serious incident where the team will reflect on what happened and will discuss their thoughts and feelings in relation to that specific incident. Whilst this is beneficial and should occur following incidents, we should be embedding team and group clinical supervision as a standard part of working. Research shows that frequent, peer-led, group clinical supervision is valued by clinical staff (Tuck, 2017). One reason for this is that a key focus of clinical supervision, whether individual or group supervision, should be to address and manage stress and to hopefully alleviate burnout (Turner and Hill, 2011). Clinical supervision is recognised as being core and crucial to clinical work by the Nursing and Midwifery Council (NMC) and the Royal College of Nurses (RCN) (Tuck, 2017). Due to this, all clinical supervision should be protected time (Sheppard, Stacey and Aubeeluck, 2018).

Regular supervision is felt to be most valuable by clinicians when it is well structured (Turner and Hill, 2011). The most frequently applied supervision model in clinical practice is Proctor's 1986 model (Sheppard, Stacey and Aubeeluck, 2018). In Proctor's model (1986), there are three key functions of supervision and those are that it should be 'normative', 'formative' and 'restorative' (Bowles and Young, 1999).

Proctor's model of clinical supervision

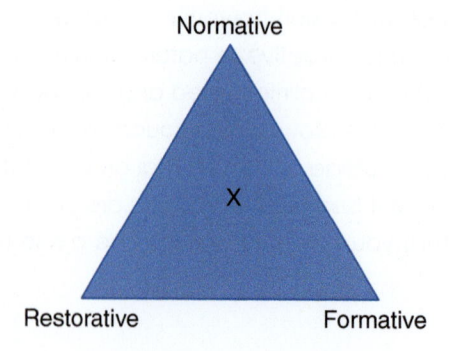

Normative

X

Restorative   Formative

As you can see in the image above, the three key features of Proctor's model can be visualised as a triangle; if all aspects are given equal weighting within a supervision, then it would be represented by the 'X' in the centre of the triangle. A clinical supervision however may not equally weigh all aspects, and within a supervision arrangement, there should be agreements between the supervisor and supervisee including the distinction between line management supervision and clinical supervision (Bowles and Young, 1999). If both supervisee and supervisor are familiar with the model, it can help to aide discussions as to what balance the supervisee would benefit from most; there should always be features of all three components, but an individual may require more of one than the other as discussed below.

'Normative' supervision would include the more traditionally understood 'line management' supervision requirements such as how the supervisee is performing within their role, do they feel they have the tools to perform the tasks required? How is their case load? Do they feel they are progressing with each client or are there any particular clients they would like to discuss? 'Formative' supervision is about the supervisee's development. What do they think their developmental needs? Do they need support to achieve these? Are there any aspects of the role that they are struggling with? This is the area in which we would consider any additional training or learning needs. 'Restorative' supervision is focussed on the supervisee's wellbeing and emotions. How are they feeling? Have there been any upsetting or distressing incidents recently? Are they feeling emotionally well? Do they feel stressed or burned out? Giving a supervisee the time and space to express their feelings is incredibly important, particularly in the field of mental health as there is so much about the work that is emotionally challenging. A good supervisor can recognise when someone is starting to struggle or feel burned out, and if they do recognise that, they should prioritise the needs of the person rather than the service which is obviously sometimes easier said than done. I have told many colleagues that they need to take a break, which may only be a few days, but when someone is starting to struggle with burnout, they will need to take a break sooner or later and later usually means for longer and is associated with much greater difficulties for the individual.

When we consider the balance of the three requirements, the 'X' would move in the triangle. Whenever I start a new supervision arrangement, I show (or usually draw) the supervisee the diagram above and explain each aspect before asking where they think they sit within the triangle. This can change each supervision session, but it really does help me as a supervisor to know what that individual specifically feels they need from me. Each individual will need a different balance, but a good supervision should always include all aspects of Proctor's model. Different people will need different balances, but you will see that there are trends. Those who are new to their roles or the profession may need a stronger focus on formative and restorative, whereas those who have been in their clinical roles for a long time and are well settled may have more of a focus on 'normative'.

Activities

Reflective Activity

Take some time to consider the diagram of Proctor's model above. Reflect on your current feelings and think about where you feel you are within the triangle in terms of your needs. Do you have a clinical supervisor at this time? If so, how comfortable do you feel in communicating this to your current supervisor? If not, think about someone who you feel you could discuss this with, they don't have to be from your clinical area, but they could be. Consider approaching them and asking them to be your clinical supervisor, and if they agree, show them the diagram above and explain your thoughts and feelings about your supervision needs and how you feel they can help you.

Case Studies

Case Study 1

Jeanette is an experienced nurse who has been working in similar clinical environments for the past 30 years. She is well liked by the team and viewed as a supportive and caring colleague who dedicates a lot of time and effort to supporting less experienced members of the team. Her clinical work has always been of a very high standard, and clients respond well to her. Jeanette has approached you as her clinical supervisor and reports that she is feeling bored and burned out. She said that for the first time in her career, she feels like she just doesn't care anymore and dreads coming to work.

What are your thoughts about how to support Jeanette as her supervisor? What aspects of Proctor's model do you feel need to take priority? Take some time to reflect on this before moving on to the suggestions below.

Answer

Jeanette is clearly struggling and there could be many reasons for this. It is important as her supervisor to give her the time and space to open up and share what she is feeling. For this, we would prioritise 'Restorative' supervision within Proctor's model. Jeanette reflects that she feels everything has become repetitive and she doesn't feel challenged anymore in this clinical environment and this is causing her frustration. Once she has reflected on and expressed this, we could focus on 'Formative' supervision as Jeanette clearly needs a new challenge or direction. We could suggest she applies for a promotion or moves to a different clinical area; although her expertise will surely be missed in her current role, Jeanette's wellbeing is more important, and from what she has communicated, she needs a change. We could also suggest that Jeanette considers further education such as doing her Advanced Practice Masters or another programme that she is interested in that would challenge her more. Although restorative and formative may be our focus, we must also consider 'Normative' and reflect on Jeanette's current role, whether she is meeting all of the service requirements of her and performing her role well.

Case Study 2

Max has recently qualified as a nurse, and as you supported him during one of his placements as a student in the unit where he now works, he asked you to be his clinical supervisor. This is the first time you have performed this role and you haven't had any specific training, but you have read about Proctor's model and feel that is a good structure and approach to take. You explain this to Max, and he agrees. After 2 months in post, Max requests a supervision with you and is very distressed. He tells you he feels totally unprepared to be a nurse; he was the nurse in charge of a shift recently, and it was incredibly stressful with several incidents that he believes are his fault. He is questioning why he came into nursing and is thinking about leaving the profession to do something totally different.

What are your thoughts about how to approach this supervision with Max? Take some time to reflect on how you would talk to Max and what your focus would initially be.

Answer

Max is clearly having a crisis of confidence, one that many newly qualified nurses will experience. If I were supervising Max, although he is clearly distressed and in need of significant 'Restorative' supervision, I would actually focus first on a 'Normative' approach. I would ask Max to talk me through the shift that he feels went so badly. When he explains it step by step, it is clear that it was not due to poor leadership on his part, but it was just a very challenging shift that would have been the same whoever had have been the nurse in charge that day. I would ask Max to reflect on what he would have changed or done differently to help him reflect on the fact that none of the incidents were due to his leadership of the shift. I would also help him reflect on what he had done well in terms of managing the shift and the incidents. I would then also share with him that everyone feels like this at some point and it is very normal to feel overwhelmed, but that he must remember he did a good job, he followed all of the policies and processes and although it was very tough, he managed the shift well. Once Max has been able to reflect on his skills and attributes, then we can focus more on the formative and restorative aspects. Within his reflection, there may have been elements that Max felt under-prepared for or that he needs development in; for this, we utilise the formative approach and consider where Max can strengthen and build upon his skills, including his reflective skills so that he is able to independently recognise his strengths more easily in the future. I would then end with the restorative focus; from the previous discussions, Max would hopefully be feeling reassured that he did not do a bad job and would be feeling better, but focussing on his feelings to conclude the supervision would be a positive approach so that Max feels his feelings are important and valid.

Clinical supervision should be a supportive and positive feature of any clinician's practice. As discussed above, it should be seen as core to our roles as nurses and that time should be protected. Good supervision however does not need to be lengthy; it could be a 20-minute session each week rather than an hour every 6 weeks as most clinicians would find that easier to accommodate and prioritise, clinical supervision should ultimately suit the supervisor and the supervisee in terms of timings and locations. As nurses, when we consider the approaches of other professions such as therapists of all kinds, it seems incredulous that it is a professional requirement for all therapists to be in their own personal therapy due to the emotional challenges of their roles, but there is no such consideration for nurses. Clinical supervision is not therapy, but it can help to support the emotional needs and wellbeing of clinical staff. It is most positive when we feel comfortable in approaching someone we respect to be our clinical supervisor. When I was in clinical practice, I asked someone who had previously been my line manager to be my clinical supervisor when I moved to a different team because we had an excellent relationship, I felt I could open up to him and I valued his input and opinion significantly. He always helped me to reflect effectively, and my wellbeing was a key priority for him.

We do not have to be managers or senior nurses to provide supervision; we can offer supervision to any of our colleagues at any time. If we see a colleague isn't quite themselves or we know something challenging has happened, we can ask them if they want an ad hoc supervision; it does not need to be formal or official, and many clinicians do this because they are supportive colleagues and don't actually think of it as providing supervision. We can suggest group supervisions (if they are not already commonplace) to help the multi-disciplinary team work more cohesively and share their thoughts and feelings. This will help build empathy and make individuals feel more supported within the team. There is an understanding within Dialectical Behavioural Therapy (DBT) that there is no absolute right answer, that everyone makes mistakes and that we should, at all times, be non-judgmental and this has been found to be a positive inclusion in group supervisions (Tuck, 2017). Supporting each other and doing so in an empathetic manner can and will lead to a more cohesive team, and this can significantly help individuals to feel better supported and emotionally more resilient, which is ultimately the core outcome of clinical supervision.

References

Bowles, N. and Young, C. (1999) 'An evaluative study of clinical supervision based on proctor's three function interactive model', *Journal of Advanced Nursing*, 30(4), pp. 958–964. doi:10.1046/j.1365-2648.1999.01179.x.

Jones, S. (2023) 'Having trouble accessing clinical supervision? You are not alone', *Mental Health Practice*, 26(1), pp. 14–15. doi:10.7748/mhp.26.1.14.s6.

Proctor (1986) B. Proctor, supervision: a co-operative exercise in accountability, M. Marken, M. Payne, Enabling and Ensuring. Leicester. National Youth Bureau for Education in Youth and Community Work.

Sheppard, F., Stacey, G. and Aubeeluck, A. (2018) 'The importance, impact and influence of group clinical supervision for graduate entry nursing students', *Nurse Education in Practice*, 28, pp. 296–301. doi:10.1016/j.nepr.2017.11.015.

Tuck, J.A. (2017) 'A new approach to team clinical supervision on an acute admissions unit', *Mental Health Practice*, 20(5), pp. 24–27. doi:10.7748/mhp.2017.e1122.

Turner, J. and HILL, A. (2011) 'Implementing clinical supervision (part 2): Using proctor's model to structure the implementation of clinical supervision in a ward setting' *Mental Health Nursing (Online)*, 31(4), pp. 14–19.

White, E. and Winstanley, J. (2021) 'Clinical supervision provided to mental health nurses in England', *British Journal of Mental Health Nursing*, 10(2), pp. 1–11. doi:10.12968/bjmh.2020.0052.

CHAPTER 21

Professional Development

One of the most amazing things about mental health nursing is just how broad the field is. There are so many different career opportunities and pathways that you will never be bored. It can be very challenging deciding where you would like to work, which area you would like to specialise in and how to develop your skills and career after becoming a mental health nurse. Mental health nurses work across all ages and so we work with mothers and babies in perinatal specialisms, children and young people in child and adolescent mental health services, working age adults between 18 and 65 and older adults that are 65+. Mental health nurses also work across all health and social care arenas including in primary care (in General Practitioner (GP) surgeries), community specialist services, the charity sector, the private sector, inpatient services, police stations, courts, prisons, youth offending teams and education. It is really incredible how broad the role can be, and if you haven't considered roles outside inpatient wards, then now is your opportunity to think about if there are any other specialisms that you are interested in moving into.

'Professional Development' is about gaining new skills and expertise as well as career development (Parsons, 2023) and that could be through formal training that is accredited or less formal means such as mentoring others or being mentored. Lack of professional and career development opportunities has been found to be a strong factor in poor retention of staff generally (Good and Aitchison, 2022), so offering options and opportunities for development is in the interest of an organisation. The current generations that are entering the workforce have higher expectations of the organisation that they are working for and will ultimately leave if they are not satisfied (Good and Aitchison, 2022), and this appears to be a significant cultural shift as previous generations tended to remain within the same organisation and seek more linear progression by promotions than the younger generations entering the field. Research has found that an individual's experiences in the workplace, both professional and social, have a significant impact on their career and retention in that environment (Kinghorn et al., 2023). Professional development can also improve confidence, which then improves satisfaction and overall performance (Parsons, 2023) which leads to better patient care, improved morale and retention

Thriving in Mental Health Nursing, First Edition. Laura Duncan.
© 2025 John Wiley & Sons Ltd. Published 2025 by John Wiley & Sons Ltd.

of staff. Any nurse's intention to continue in a role is strongly connected to their job satisfaction and professional confidence within that role (Kinghorn et al., 2023), and studies have identified that although burnout may be more prevalent in the medical profession, nurses tend to consider leaving their profession much more frequently (Hämmig 2018) which highlights the importance of improving morale. Professional development is important for potential career advancement and promotions (Parsons, 2023), but feeling as though you are learning and improving your knowledge and skills is key to overall job (and life) satisfaction. In summary, professional development needs to be an organisational priority as supporting staff to grow, learn and improve has direct benefits to not only the individual staff member but also to clients and the team they work within. You are also much more likely to retain staff if they feel well supported and they have opportunities available to them.

Activity

Take some time to think about where you would like to be in your career in 10 years' time:

- Do you want to be working in inpatient services and doing shifts or would you prefer a more 9–5 based role?
- Would you like to be managing a team?
- Is there a particular client group you want to work with?
- Are there any new areas of nursing that you are interested in?
- Would you like to teach or train others?
- Would you like to undertake any courses such as advanced practice, non-medical prescribing, teaching or leadership?
- What is important to you in terms of work/life balance?

There may be several things you are unsure of, but for most people, if the question is 'Do you want to be working in the same role, in the same environment in 10 years?', then there would usually be a fairly quick and strong response. Either 'Yes! I love my job and can't see myself ever leaving!' or 'No, I couldn't stay here another 10 years!'. If the answer is no, then you need to spend some real time reflecting on where you would like to be instead. The important thing to remember in nursing is that, as discussed above, you are never stuck. If you aren't happy in a particular role or style of working, it may be a challenge, you may need to think about upskilling or additional training/qualifications, but you can always move to somewhere that you will enjoy more and that will be a better fit for you.

Many people are interested in career development and advancement in the context of being promoted in either the same or a similar clinical environment. If you are thinking about career advancement, then you will at some point need to consider applications and interviews. Even if you are not thinking about your next career steps in terms of moving role, as registered nurses we must all complete 'Revalidation' every three years (NMC, 2018) to ensure that we are safe to continue practicing. Due to this, it is good practice to consistently keep a portfolio throughout your career. It will make applications and interviews much easier to prepare for and will ensure that you have everything ready for revalidation when you need it. A professionally prepared portfolio can help to illustrate your experience and expertise as a nurse

(Oermann, 2002) and is a way to showcase all of your skills (Khan, 2023). Portfolios can help to provide evidence of meeting competencies and requirements for not only revalidation, but appraisals as well (Oermann, 2002).

There are many different ways you could structure your portfolio, but key areas that you should consider including are:

- A 'This is me' section – This could be a '1 page profile' for yourself, or your CV but include some personal details that make you 'you' such as your hobbies and interests.
- An education/training section – Keep all of your certificates, diplomas and achievements in this section; it keeps them safe and together for whenever you need them, but sometimes we can forget everything we've achieved.
- A 'Feedback' section – Keep feedback from clients, colleagues and managers all in one place. This is a really important section and is often overlooked. Feedback is incredibly important, and negative feedback can help us to develop further, but positive feedback can help us to recognise our own skills and knowledge. Feedback is also crucial for revalidation, so keeping it in a single place is very helpful.
- A 'Personal Development Plan' – This should be something very personalised to you; you could write it in the form of a reflection or use a more structured approach in terms of considering where you would like to go next and how you plan to achieve that, whatever 'development' means to you.

Another way of thinking about a potential structure for a portfolio is; 'this is who I am, where I've been and where I'm going'. Portfolios can help to provide evidence of meeting competencies and requirements for not only revalidation but for annual appraisals as well (Oermann, 2002). It is important though to remember that a portfolio needs to be focussed and highlight your accomplishment and skills rather than simply being an accumulation of every piece of paper throughout your career (Oermann, 2002).

The next key consideration within professional development is completing applications and interviews. Job applications in the healthcare sector can be very challenging as each application is unique and will have slightly different formats and requirements. An application can require extensive amounts of information that demonstrate you have the required knowledge, skills and expertise for the role (Sole, 2012); however, it is crucial to ensure that you are providing this information in a clear and concise manner. Many people do not fully recognise that a good application is key to securing an interview and therefore do not give this stage the attention that it requires (Potterton, 2011). As nurses, we can sometimes feel more confident communicating verbally and 'selling' ourselves at interview, but ultimately, if your application is not of a good standard, you are unlikely to be offered an interview (Sole, 2012).

Key considerations for completing a job application:

- Take your time! It can feel very high pressure; particularly, if the closing date is soon, but even if you only have a few hours, you can still take enough time to produce an excellent application.
- Pay attention to the role you are applying for. If you are actively looking for a new job, you may be submitting several applications for different roles and services. Make sure you are looking carefully at the person specification for each role you apply for and are ensuring your application is tailored to each application. Some sections such as your personal information and education will of course be the same/similar, but the supporting information section will not be.

- Read the person specification carefully. If the essential criteria contain a qualification that you don't possess, consider whether this is a suitable role for you. If you are unclear or unsure, contact the person named on the advert to discuss with them. Ultimately, if the role requires someone with an Advanced Practice Masters and you don't have one and aren't currently working towards that qualification, you are unlikely to be shortlisted, so you are ultimately going to be disappointed. If you contact the named person and they say that they would accept someone who is willing to undertake that qualification, then that means that you can simply include in your supporting information that you would want to undertake that qualification.
- Be critical of your own skills, do you think you are the right person for this role? If you can't confidently say 'yes', then reconsider whether it is an appropriate role for you at this time.
- Consider your transferrable skills. You may have previous employment outside of healthcare that you feel isn't relevant, but there are likely to be many transferrable skills such as communication, handling difficult situations, leadership, line management, etc., that are very transferrable. Just ensure that you are making it very clear how these are transferrable to the role you are applying for within your application.
- Use the person specification to help you structure your supporting information section, if you work through it and include your evidence and experience of how you meet each 'essential' criterion and hopefully most of the 'desirable' criteria, you can be confident you have addressed each point effectively and will feel more confident you will be shortlisted for interview. It is important to remember that if you do not make it clear that you meet all of the 'essential' criteria in your application, you are unlikely to be shortlisted.
- Remember it isn't just a 'tick box' exercise. It can be very difficult when you are ensuring you communicate how you meet the person specification, but you also need to communicate your passion, enthusiasm and personality as well. You ultimately want the person shortlisting to read your application and feel like they have a good picture of you and are excited to meet with you for interview.
- Proof read! Many job application websites don't have spell check or grammar checking facilities, so it is helpful to use another application such as Microsoft Word to write your application and ask someone else to proof read for you if you are not confident. Communication is a key skill within all healthcare roles, so submitting an application with lots of errors and mistakes does not show that you have excellent communication skills; therefore, be very mindful of this when writing your application!

The next stage in changing role is the job interview. This can be a nerve-wracking and daunting experience, regardless of how experienced and confident you are! The key to feeling confident walking in to a job interview is preparation. Preparing effectively by researching the role and organisation you are applying for is crucial for any job interview (Evans, 2022). Depending on the role you are applying for, the questions you could be asked could be very broad ranging. Many health and social care organisations have moved towards a 'values-based' interview approach. Values-based interviews are focussed on establishing whether key personality traits that are core to good patient care and the organisation are present in the individual and these traits commonly include empathy, care, compassion and equality (McGuire et al., 2016). We have moved away from focussing purely on skills, and employers now feel that someone would be a 'good fit' for their team if they treat clients with dignity, respect, kindness and compassion.

Key considerations for a job interview:

- Dress appropriately. Do not wear sportswear or anything dirty/with holes in it, etc. You want to make a good first impression, and looking presentable is key for this. It can be difficult when you are used to wearing either a uniform or more casual clothes, but dress to impress at an interview.
- Smile! When you are nervous, it can be difficult, but you want the panel to think you are warm, friendly and personable, so be conscious of your body language including smiling, eye contact and how you are sitting. Practice at home how you will sit and how you will walk in to the panel. Decide before hand if you want to shake the hand of each panel member or not as making that decision in the moment can fluster you and make you feel awkward.
- When you have sat down, say that it is nice to meet them all or thank them for seeing you, it shows that you are polite and demonstrates that you respect their time as well, it is a positive way to start the interview as well. Acknowledge if you are feeling very nervous, an interview panel understands that the process can be intimidating and nerve wracking, so acknowledging that you are feeling nervous can give the panel the opportunity to reassure you.
- Take in water with you. It can be easy to get flustered in an interview environment, and nerves can mean you get a dry mouth. Taking a sip of water after a question is asked gives you a chance to formulate your response in your head before you start speaking as well.
- Keep your responses focussed. It is very easy to go on a tangent and not actually answer the question! There are lots of different ways to do this, but one helpful tactic is the 'STAR' approach where your response is structured as: Situation, Task, Action and Result. This approach also ensures that you are giving the full picture of a scenario with the outcome of your actions as well.
- Say 'I'! You may have been part of a team who performed the task you are talking about, but take credit for your role and participation. Many people struggle to acknowledge their own actions effectively, so ensure that you are being clear about what you specifically did in any given situation.
- Have key experiences prepared. You are likely to be asked about situations that involved you demonstrating leadership, resilience or a service/quality improvement, so have your answers prepared in advance. Think also about your core values and skills, what would you like the panel to know about you by the time you leave?
- Reflect back to the panel. Many questions in interviews are detailed and sometimes have several components to them. It can be very easy to not fully address each aspect of these questions in particular and so a good technique to use when you have finished your response is to ask the panel 'Does that fully answer your question?', 'Have I covered each aspect of the question appropriately?' or 'Have I provided enough depth and detail?'. This will also give you an idea of how the interview is going and give the panel the opportunity to ask for clarity or further explanation. If the panel says 'You've answered everything thoroughly', then you can be more confident moving forward to the next question.
- Have questions prepared for the end of the interview. They could be practical questions about the role itself or where the team feel the service could be developed further. It shows interest and engagement in the team and service, but aim to ask at least two questions at the end of the interview. Have them written on a notepad in front of you if you feel you may forget or go blank at the end of the interview!

- When leaving, thank the panel for their time and say that you are looking forward to hearing from them. Ensure that you leave on a positive and warm note.
- Seek feedback. If you are unsuccessful, ask for feedback and although disappointing, this can help you with future applications and interviews.

Professional development is an important area to consider throughout your career, and taking time to think about where you want to be and what you want to be doing is vital to ensure your wellbeing and satisfaction in your career. Reflecting on what interests you and what is important to you in your work life can lead to finding roles that you thrive in and enjoy. Making the decision that you would like to change or move role can be daunting; particularly, if it comes out of being unsatisfied or unhappy in your current work, but if you use your reflective skills and explore your options thoroughly, it should be an exciting step to take. Keeping a well-structured and organised portfolio can help you to identify your strengths and expertise in preparation for a promotion or role change. Applications and interviews can be very challenging and difficult, particularly, if you are unsuccessful, but it is always a learning opportunity, so ask for feedback and reflect on what you did well as well as what you could improve for next time. Sometimes you can perform excellently at interview but just not be the right fit for the role, and that is ultimately the better outcome for you as well. It is a hard and draining process, but if you are looking to move into a different area or team, be persistent and the right role will happen in time.

References

Evans, N. (2022) 'Band 7 roles: Is it time you stepped up to the next level?', *Cancer Nursing Practice*, 21(4), pp. 12–13. doi:10.7748/cnp.21.4.12.s5.

Good, V.S. and Atchison, J. (2022) 'What's my next step? Navigating nursing career progression', *Nursing Management*, 53(12), pp. 12–19. doi:10.1097/01.numa.0000897452.96484.20.

Hämmig, O. (2018) 'Explaining burnout and the intention to leave the profession among health professionals – A cross-sectional study in a hospital setting in Switzerland', *BMC Health Services Research*, 18(1). doi:10.1186/s12913-018-3556-1.

Khan, R. (2023) *Tips for developing your professional portfolio*. Nursing Times. Available at: https://www.nursingtimes.net/students/tips-for-developing-your-professional-portfolio-03-01-2023/ (Accessed: 8 March 2024).

Kinghorn, G. et al. (2023) 'Why do nurses seek employment in forensic mental health and what are their first impressions of the clinical environment? A mixed methods study', *Journal of Advanced Nursing*, 79(9), pp. 3622–3631. doi:10.1111/jan.15703.

McGuire, C. et al. (2016) 'Improving the quality of the NHS workforce through values and competency-based selection', *Nursing Management*, 23(4), pp. 26–33. doi:10.7748/nm.2016.e1502.

Nursing and Midwifery Council (NMC) (2018) *The code: Professional standards of practice and behaviour for nurses, midwives and nursing associates*. London: NMC.

Oermann, M.H. (2002) 'Developing a professional portfolio in nursing', *Orthopaedic Nursing*, 21(2), pp. 73–78. doi:10.1097/00006416-200203000-00013.

Parsons, L. (2023) *Why is professional development important? – Professional & executive development: Harvard DCE, Professional & Executive Development|Harvard DCE*. Available at: https://professional.dce.harvard.edu/blog/why-is-professional-development-important/ (Accessed: 8 March 2024).

Potterton, J. (2011) 'NHS job applications: a guide for nursing students', *Nursing Standard (through 2013)*, 25(46), pp. 42–47; quiz 48.

Sole, V. (2012) 'Job applications', *Nursing Standard (through 2013)*, 26(19), p. 57.

CHAPTER 22

Social Determinants of Health Chapter

The way and conditions in which people live impact their health and wellbeing, the external factors that influence this are commonly referred to as 'The Social Determinants of Health' and can include the economic, social and political landscape around an individual (Mwoka et al., 2021). One of the most stark examples of this is that there is a widening life expectancy gap that is strongly correlated to increasing poverty levels (White et al., 2018). This means that in the United Kingdom, poorer people die younger than rich people and the 'wealth gap' has become an increasingly important topic of conversation over recent years. It has also been established that males who experience social and economic hardship are more likely to die prematurely (White et al., 2018). Children from low-income households are believed to have an increased rate of physical and mental health issues with poor mental health and wellbeing in childhood and adolescence being correlated to difficulties in adulthood including in employment, education and relationships (Fitzsimons et al., 2017). The Covid-19 pandemic is believed to have exacerbated socio-economic health inequalities such as poor/unstable employment and housing (Lombardo et al., 2023). Since the start of the Covid-19 pandemic, there have been increased rates of anxiety, depression, loneliness, poorer sleep, self-injurious behaviour and abuse in the United Kingdom with those who had the poorest levels of mental health and wellbeing pre-pandemic experiencing the most significant worsening of their mental health during the lockdown periods in particular (Lombardo et al., 2023).

Poor quality, unsafe or unstable housing has a clear impact on someone's health, and homelessness is a significant issue in the United Kingdom with 70% of young homeless people having mental health issues, and those with mental health issues are twice as likely to become homeless as the general population (Mwoka et al., 2021). Homelessness can be the factor that causes a significant deterioration in someone's mental health, but it can also work the other way, with mental health causing or contributing to someone becoming homeless. In the United Kingdom, housing prices and costs have risen significantly more than incomes over the past 40 years which means

Thriving in Mental Health Nursing, First Edition. Laura Duncan.
© 2025 John Wiley & Sons Ltd. Published 2025 by John Wiley & Sons Ltd.

that younger or lower income individuals have found housing to be unaffordable which has a significant influence on someone's mental health and wellbeing (Mwoka et al., 2021). Healthcare professionals have an important role to play in improving public health (Graham, 2018), and without improving the social determinants of health, overall population health is unlikely to improve (Mwoka et al., 2021). Many factors that play into the social determinants of health can become a vicious cycle, and one of the starkest examples of this is that having poor health can lead to job loss and unemployment, but poor working environments can also lead to poor health (Sewdas et al., 2019).

One of the clearest models and explanations of how social and economic factors influence health and wellbeing is that of Dahlgren and Whitehead (Dahlgren and Whitehead, 2021). The original model, sometimes referred to as 'The Rainbow Model', was commissioned by the World Health Organisation in 1991 but was rejected for being 'too complicated' before it was then published separately in 1991 and adopted by the King's fund in 1993 which led to it becoming recognised prominently within the United Kingdom and later internationally (Dahlgren and Whitehead, 2021). One of the key benefits of the model was that it enabled sectors outside of healthcare to understand their role and importance in improving health inequalities across the population (Dahlgren and Whitehead, 2021). The most recent version of the model can be seen below:

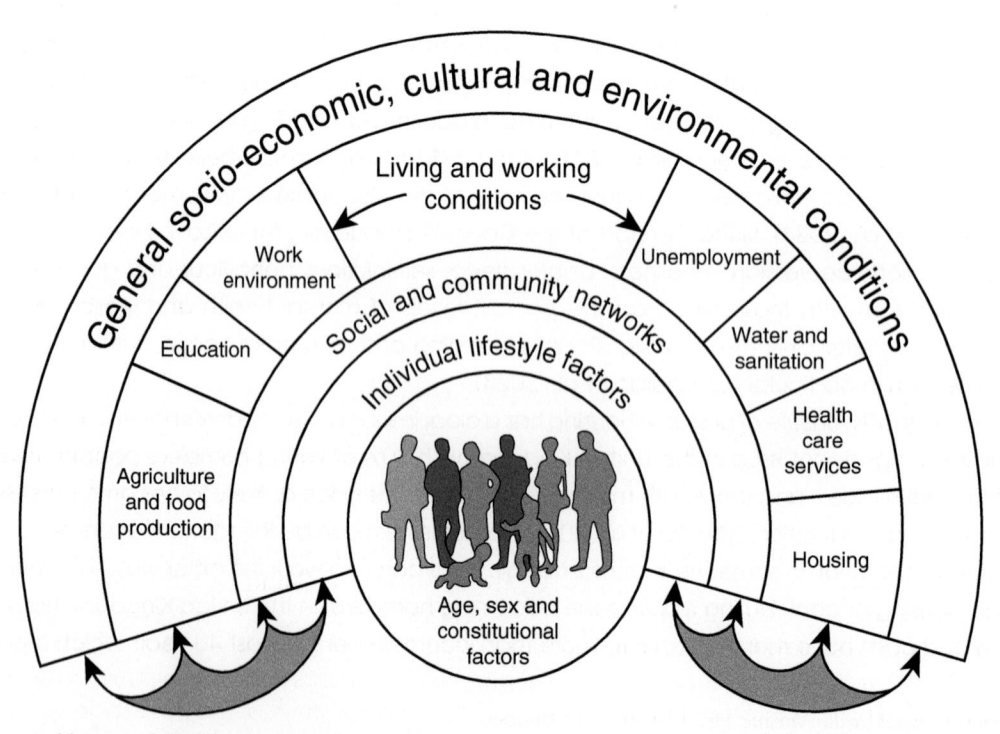

Source: Dahlgren et al. (2021)/with permission of Elsevier.

At the centre of the model, we see the people and the factors that cannot be changed such as their age and genetic factors. The next layer is then the 'individual lifestyle factors', and this will include personal choices such as smoking, diet and exercise levels. 'Social and Community Networks' are important and, as the arrows below the rainbow indicate, influence our lifestyle factors and choices. Having access to safe, green spaces and friends who enjoy jogging will mean you may be more likely to take up jogging than if your social circle do not enjoy exercise and you live in a built up environment with no access to green spaces to exercise in an enjoyable manner. The next layer is 'Living and Working Conditions', and we will explore how each of these could impact health and wellbeing via individual case studies below. 'General socio-economic, cultural and environmental conditions' relate to the bigger picture for the population including factors such as air pollution, access to healthcare and education in that society.

Agriculture and Food Production Case Study

In a country that is experiencing severe weather events such as drought or flooding, this will have a significant impact on how much food can be produced and how sustainable food production is. This will mean there is less availability at the individual level for fresh food produced locally. It will also mean that prices are likely to increase, causing those who are socio-economically disadvantaged to make difficult choices. Many of us will have seen clearly that there were food shortages in the United Kingdom during the Covid-19 pandemic with supermarket shelves being empty of certain foods, but there have also been shortages of various fruits and vegetables including potatoes in recent years due to agricultural issues. For Jenny who has a family of five to feed on a limited income, the choice of fresh and healthy options has become increasingly difficult, meaning she relies on low budget options such as pasta to feed her family. While pasta is not an unhealthy choice, not having a balanced meal with protein and vegetables as well as pasta could lead to malnutrition, which can then lead to the development of health issues.

Education Case Study

Education has a long lasting impact on an individual that can be difficult to truly understand when key educational decisions are made. It is now mandatory for all under 18s to be in education of some form in the United Kingdom, but whether someone engages with their education is a very different matter. Johnny hated school and began truanting when he was a teenager; he then did not sit his GCSE exams and so therefore could not study A Levels, and he agreed to undertake a T Level qualification but did not attend or submit any of his assignments. Johnny made all of these decisions before he was legally considered an adult, but now, not having any qualifications means his choice of job options is very limited. If Johnny wanted to go to university, he would have to re-do GCSEs and A Levels to meet the entry requirements which depending on his living situation may not be possible if he also needs to work to support himself. Because of his poor educational attainment, Johnny works in low-paying manual jobs, which will be discussed in the next case study.

Work Environment Case Study

Poor working environments have long been known to have negative effects on an individual's long term health. Asbestos is a good example of this as it was widely used in buildings for construction, and it was not until 1999 that it was banned from use. If someone was working in construction and using asbestos regularly, inhaling asbestos dust can cause lung cancer, so for those individuals, their work could directly cause lung cancer. In poor working environments, we also see an increased risk of musculo-skeletal issues and injuries; these can then cause reduced mobility either due to loss of function or ongoing pain, which negatively impacts activity levels which can increase the risk of obesity and then associated health conditions. Experiencing chronic pain is also strongly associated with lower levels of wellbeing generally and can lead to the development of mental health issues such as anxiety and depression. Physically strenuous jobs are not the only ones that can have a negative impact on our health; office and desk-based roles where you are sedentary for much of the day can be just as dangerous for your health, and shift working has been repeatedly proven to have a negative long-term effect on health. Johnny has limited choices when it comes to employment and has been working as a delivery driver for several different food delivery apps. Johnny can have his shifts cancelled at very short notice if there is limited demand for drivers, and sometimes he can work long hours for much less than minimum wage. Johnny feels very stressed as he does not know how to obtain a more stable job that is safer than riding a bike on busy roads and he spends significant amounts of time worrying about being able to pay his rent and bills. Johnny sleeps very little because of financial worries, and his mood has been getting worse and worse. Having stable and safe employment is crucial to our overall wellbeing, and we can see from Johnny's example the negative impact on wellbeing that poor quality or unstable employment can have.

Unemployment Case Study

At the time of writing, Universal Credit is less than £400 per month for a single adult over the age of 25. Even if rent is covered by additional housing benefits, £400 for all bills a month is difficult to manage. When you consider gas, electricity, water, council tax, etc., it seems that £400 would probably leave you with less than £50 per week for food and groceries. This would work out as around £2.40 per meal, which although that is achievable does not leave much capacity for fresh fruits, vegetables, meat or fish, meaning that someone's diet could become nutritionally poor very quickly. We see frequent headlines around people having to choose whether to 'heat or eat', parents not eating so that their children can and that there are now over 2500 food banks in the United Kingdom. Unemployment not only impacts your housing, heating and food, but it is a stressor within itself which can increase negative thoughts, low mood, depression and anxiety and is associated with lower life expectancy overall. Long-term unemployment is bad for not only physical health but also your mental health. Siruti has had respiratory issues since childhood and now has emphysema and requires oxygen therapy. Due to this, Siruti struggles to leave the house independently as she becomes fatigued very quickly. She has been unable to find a job that she can reliably engage with and has found even remote working from home to be very challenging due to her condition and has now been unemployed for four years. Siruti spends most of her time alone at home and feels very isolated. She has no money left after paying all of her bills and for groceries to be delivered as she cannot go to the supermarket herself. Siruti used to enjoy seeing her friends, but she cannot afford to join in the activities they suggest, and slowly she has stopped hearing from them. Siruti has felt low in mood for a very long time and has stopped completing activities like showering or cleaning her home. Siruti has started noticing she has a skin issue, but she does not feel like going to the doctor and leaves it to worsen. Siruti feels constantly bored and does not have any social network that she can talk to. In this example, we can see how unemployment has negatively impacted Siruti's quality of life and how quickly someone's health and wellbeing can deteriorate when they have limited means and social support.

Water and Sanitation Case Study

Not having access to clean water and sanitation can have very serious and immediate health consequences. Not having access to suitable drinking water can cause severe dehydration but also increase the likelihood of contracting water-borne infections/diseases such as dysentery, typhoid, E. Coli and Salmonella and can also cause diarrhoea and vomiting. Poor sanitation can also cause significant health issues including skin problems/infections, respiratory issues, dental problems and gastro-intestinal issues. For women, not having access to appropriate sanitation facilities during menstruation can be particularly dangerous as not changing sanitary products or being able to clean them appropriately can lead to toxic shock syndrome and even sepsis, which is immediately and urgently life threatening. Those who are homeless are much less likely to have access to safe and appropriate sanitation facilities, but poor quality housing can also lead to poor sanitation conditions in the home. In the United Kingdom, it is illegal for a water company to cut off your supply of water, even if you have not paid your water bill, but water provision issues and sanitation issues disproportionately affect the socio-economically disadvantaged and poorest in society. Sasha is 14 years old, and her family is struggling to make ends meet. Sasha has been unable to buy sanitary product during her menstruation and has been using rags made from old t-shirts. She is hand washing these between use, but she is embarrassed for her family to know and has been hiding them, and they have not been drying thoroughly. Sasha spends her day at school worrying about whether they will provide adequate protection or whether she will bleed through her underwear and uniform as this has happened before. Sasha is at increased risk of developing infections or toxic shock syndrome and she is unable to concentrate on her lessons in school meaning she is falling behind. She is too embarrassed to talk to anyone about her situation, so she has started isolating herself from her friends. We can understand that this is going to have a negative impact on Sasha's mental health and general wellbeing, but it is also at risk of seriously damaging her physical health.

Healthcare Services Case Study

In the United Kingdom, we have the National Health Service (NHS) which is free at the point of access, which means that you can ultimately have almost any illness or ailment treated with little to no cost. If you have a chronic condition and disability, are under 18 (or in full-time education) or are in receipt of benefits, then you will also not pay for prescriptions, and for those who do pay for prescriptions, they are capped so that they are affordable for most who are in employment. Dentistry is slightly different where you will normally pay for an appointment and follow-up procedures if needed, but again there are caps to this and those in receipt of benefits such as Universal Credit will be exempted. This means that for the majority of the population, appropriate healthcare is available, but the key issue that we face in the United Kingdom currently is waiting lists. For those who can afford privatised healthcare, waiting lists become much less of an issue, so again being poor means you have less options and are forced to wait until the NHS can address your issue. We also hear the term 'postcode lottery' quite frequently in the United Kingdom, and this is because the same level and availability of services is not equal in all parts of the country. Availability of services is a much more significant issue in rural areas in particular, but entitlement to services such as fertility services and in-vitro fertilisation can vary widely across the United Kingdom. There is also significant regional variability in General Practitioner (GP) provision and social care provision. Jack is a retired farmer living in the rural South East of England. He lives alone and has no family in the area. He stepped on an old nail in an outhouse 2 days ago and initially dismissed it as 'just a scratch'. It has been becoming more swollen, red, hot to the touch and painful. Jack can no longer walk on his foot as it has become so sore. He calls his GP but is told that he must call back at 8 am the next day, which he does. He asks for a home visit because he cannot drive to the surgery with his foot in so much pain, and the GP receptionist advises that unfortunately, there is no availability for home visits as Jack lives so far from the surgery; none of the practice staff would be able to attend that day due to how busy they are. Jack hangs up and is very frustrated. Throughout the day, his foot becomes more and more painful; he calls 111, and they advise he needs to attend the hospital. As Jack cannot drive himself and has no one that could drive him there, he calls for an ambulance, but as it is deemed 'non-urgent', it takes several hours for the ambulance to arrive. Jack is eventually admitted to the hospital, and the infection in his foot at this point is very severe. He is admitted for three days and is fit enough to be discharged from hospital, but as there is no social services support available at that time, Jack must remain in hospital until he can mobilise fully independently which takes an additional two weeks. As we can see in this example, if there had have been better provision for the GP surgery, Jack may not have required hospitalisation in the first place, and if there had have been improved social services provision in his area, he may have been discharged home much quicker.

Housing Case Study

Housing is becoming an increasingly difficult area within the United Kingdom. The homeless population is continuously rising, and even for those with some form of housing, this is frequently not up to the standard that would be deemed safe or acceptable. For those living in unsafe areas or 'emergency accommodation', this can frequently feel dangerous which would have a clear and significant impact on your mood and stress levels. Many homes in the United Kingdom also experience damp and mould which can be very challenging to treat or manage safely. Living in a damp and mouldy home can significantly increase the risk of respiratory conditions and can even lead to pneumonia. If someone is admitted to a hospital and treated for pneumonia and then they are discharged home to a mould-ridden home, they will likely become unwell again and require further hospitalisations. Those living in cramped and overcrowded living conditions are also at increased risk of infection and disease as they will spread more quickly when people are living in such close proximity. Shanise and Shaun have a four-week-old baby. They have been living in social housing for several years, and in their current flat, there is a significant mould problem. They have reported this to their local housing authority who advised it was not significant enough for them to be moved elsewhere, and they advised this is because they had been attempting to clean and treat it. They were left with no option but to leave the mould to grow, so the housing authority would understand the seriousness of it and move them to a more appropriate property. They are now living with their new baby in a flat where there is black mould from floor to ceiling on every wall, the curtains are mouldy and they are struggling to keep their clothes, and the baby's clothes free of mould. They are distraught at having to live in this environment but feel they have no choice but to leave it to worsen, so they can be moved. The baby is breathing in mould every day, and the consequences of this on their ongoing health, even into adulthood, could be dire.

As we can see from these case studies, each aspect of the Dahlgren and Whitehead Model (2021) can individually have a significant impact on not only physical health but mental health and well-being as well. Many of these factors interplay against each other, and for those living in the most socio-economically disadvantaged areas, they can be negatively impacted by several, if not all, of the components simultaneously. When we understand what 'social determinants of health' are, we can then start considering how they can be addressed and improved and possibly the most impactful work around addressing social inequalities came from 'The Marmot Review: Fair Society, Healthy Lives' (Marmot, 2010).

The Marmot review (Marmot, 2010) was a seminal report examining the role of social inequalities on health and giving guidance on how to minimise and improve these throughout the United Kingdom. Marmot (2010) found that the lower someone's social status, the worse their health is. The Marmot review (2010) states that:

'Reducing health inequalities will require action on six policy objectives:

- Give every child the best start in life
- Enable all children, young people and adults to maximise their capabilities and have control over their lives
- Create fair employment and good work for all
- Ensure healthy standards of living for all
- Create and develop healthy and sustainable communities
- Strengthen the role and impact of ill health prevention' (Marmot, 2010 p. 15).

The need to ensure that all children are given the 'best start in life' should be clear to all, but many will believe that that is already happening. The need of having a 'good start' in childhood cannot be overstated as good school performance impacts educational attainment, which impacts career opportunities, which impacts living conditions throughout adulthood (Marmot, 2020). The importance of improving health through addressing social inequalities is summarised by Marmot as 'Social justice is a matter of life and death' (Marmot, 2010 p. 34). Ultimately, many health inequalities are absolutely avoidable, so that is why it becomes a social justice issue as I do not believe anyone would say it is 'fair' or 'right' that a child who is born to a poor family in a socio-economically deprived area should have more health issues and die younger than someone born to a wealthy family in an affluent area. Ten years on from the original Marmot review, the government policy of austerity has led to significant increases in child poverty, reduced funding for education, increased use of food banks due to families being unable to afford basic necessities and a housing crisis (Marmot, 2020). Life expectancy has historically consistently improved, but after 2011, this slowed significantly, and for women living in socio-economically deprived areas in the North of England, life expectancy has actually started decreasing (Marmot, 2020). The key message is that health is not only about healthcare services but also the environment and conditions in which people live (Marmot, 2020).

As we have established, the social determinants of health contribute significantly to health inequalities (Mwoka et al., 2021) and poor individual health and wellbeing outcomes. So what is the answer and what can health and social care professionals do to address this and support people who may be experiencing social inequality that could impact their health? One approach that is gaining momentum is that of 'Social Prescribing'. Social prescribing is defined as the process of connecting individuals with non-clinical services to improve their overall health and wellbeing (Alderwick et al., 2018). Social prescribing is focussed on supporting individuals to engage with non-clinical services in the community to help them with their social needs and long-term health conditions, focussing on supporting individuals with the wider social determinants of health (Wildman et al., 2019). It has existed in some forms since at least the 1960s where physicians in the Mississippi Delta region in the United States of America prescribed food to malnourished children (Alderwick et al., 2018). If a child is malnourished, the best way to address that is to improve their diet and food intake rather than by prescribing medication and so it demonstrates how logical the approach is in preventing ill health. Social prescribing can assist with a variety of needs including housing issues, benefit advice, employment or educational needs (Wildman et al., 2019) and it is proven to be evidence based and a person-centred approach that has been shown to improve wellbeing (Nowak and Mulligan, 2021). Addressing the social needs of individuals has become an increasing healthcare priority (Alderwick et al., 2018) and social prescribing has a much more holistic focus (Wildman et al., 2019). The medical model focusses on disease and illness which frequently has an underlying social cause (Nowak and Mulligan, 2021) so to effectively 'treat' an issue, we must focus more on the social influences that may be causing or worsening the condition. In the United Kingdom, we have seen the implementation of 'Social Prescribing Link Workers' in recent years with The NHS setting a target to connect at least 900,000 people with social prescribing by 2024 (Nowak and Mulligan, 2021). Social prescribing link workers provide support to individuals to understand and address behaviours that may be harming their health (such as smoking) and they work with clients with a range of health needs or risks (Wildman et al., 2019). Those who have engaged with social prescribing services generally report good levels of satisfaction and improved health and wellbeing (Alderwick et al., 2018) as a result of their engagement with social prescribing. Social Prescribing Link workers are able to work with individuals more flexibly to engage them with support or services in the community.

Social Prescribing Case Study

When I worked within The Criminal Justice System, the organisation I worked for had a 'Community Link Worker' (CLW) Team which ultimately functioned as Social Prescribing Link Workers. They received referrals from clinicians (such as myself) and worked with them on a short term basis to engage clients with appropriate teams and services in the community. One client I assessed and referred to the CLW team was 'Toby'. Toby had been incarcerated from the ages of 17–23 and upon release from prison, had been supported with housing. His benefits had been sanctioned and that meant that he wasn't receiving his full entitlement and could no longer pay his rent. He was then evicted and deemed to have made himself 'intentionally homeless' which means that the local Housing Authority had no responsibility to provide him with accommodation. He had been in a relationship and started living with his girlfriend but this relationship wasn't stable, they argued frequently and he left her and became street homeless. He had been a 'looked after child' since he was five years old and had a very limited support network. He had struggled to get identification in the form of a passport due to not having any legal documents to prove his identity. He had returned to his now ex-girlfriend's home to retrieve his passport but the interaction had become heated. He called the police to help him retrieve his passport without any further issues and as his ex-girlfriend had presented a knife at the door to threaten him, the police were intending to arrest her. Toby didn't want that to happen as he was just focussed on getting his passport and leaving and this then led to him arguing with the police, which escalated and led to him being arrested and brought into custody.

When I assessed Toby, his needs were very clear. He was homeless with no access to benefits and was not registered with a GP so could not prove links to any specific area. It was early December and the emergency winter shelters were open so I was able to arrange a bed in a shelter for the night but this was clearly a much longer term issue and need for Toby. I referred him to the CLW team and my colleague worked with him to review his benefit documentation, meaning he was then receiving a stable source of income. She also supported him with attending the Local Housing Authority and was able to obtain 'emergency housing' for him due to his level of vulnerability. This obviously addressed his most immediate needs, which was incredibly positive but the CLW didn't stop there! Due to her links and knowledge of the local area and resources available in the community, she was able to find a programme that taught someone to be a bicycle mechanic. It was a free course that led to a certificate and links to employment afterwards. She also helped him to register with a local GP service and referred him to an improved access to psychological therapy service for ongoing emotional support.

In less than two months, Toby went from being street homeless with no way of supporting himself to having a qualification and a job as well as housing. He could access healthcare because he was now registered with a GP and was going to get the support he needed to move forward with his life in a positive manner through ongoing counselling support. The impact of the social prescribing interventions led by the CLW in this case are a clear example of how important the social needs are of people to improve someone's health, wellbeing and ultimately their life. Without these interventions, Toby would likely have continued to be street homeless and his physical and mental health would have deteriorated quickly.

Being able to link people in with appropriate services and support in the community is vital in addressing health inequalities and improving the social determinants of health not only at an individual level but also across society. We see an increasing disparity in the lives and health of those from the richest and poorest areas of society which is simply not fair. As health and social care professionals, one of the best things we can do to ensure we are supporting people holistically and considering their social needs as well as their health needs is to know what is available in our local area. Take time to look into services for each core issue in social determinants of health in your area. Do you know who could help locally with housing issues, benefits advice, unemployment or educational needs? Have you got a social prescribing service in your area? Having this information to hand will help you support your clients in all aspects of their life and will have a significant impact on not only individual but overall population health and wellbeing.

References

Alderwick, H.A.J. et al. (2018) 'Social prescribing in the U.S. and England: Emerging interventions to address patients' social needs', *American Journal of Preventive Medicine*, 54(5), pp. 715–718. doi:10.1016/j.amepre.2018.01.039.

Dahlgren, G. and Whitehead, M. (2021) 'The Dahlgren-Whitehead model of health determinants: 30 years on and still chasing rainbows', *Public Health*, 199, pp. 20–24. doi:10.1016/j.puhe.2021.08.009.

Fitzsimons, E. et al. (2017) 'Poverty dynamics and parental mental health: Determinants of childhood mental health in the UK', *Social Science & Medicine (1982)*, 175, pp. 43–51. doi: 10.1016/j.socscimed.2016.12.040.

Graham, G. (2018) 'To address pressing public health issues, look Upstream The social determinants of health: Looking upstream by Kathryn Strother Ratcliff Cambridge (UK). Polity Press, 2017 256 pp., $69.95," *Health affairs (Project Hope)*, 37(3), pp. 510–510. doi:10.1377/hlthaff.2018.0085.

Lombardo, C. et al. (2023) 'Inequalities and mental health during the coronavirus pandemic in the UK: A mixed-methods exploration', *BMC Public Health*, 23(1), p. 1830. doi:10.1186/s12889-023-16523-9.

Marmot, M. (2010) *Fair society, healthy lives: The Marmot review.*

Marmot, M. (2020) 'Health equity in England: The Marmot review 10 years on', *BMJ (Clinical Research Ed.)*, 368, p. m693. doi:10.1136/bmj.m693.

Mwoka, M. et al. (2021) 'Housing as a social determinant of health: Evidence from Singapore, the UK, and Kenya: The 3-D commission,' *Journal of Urban Health: Bulletin of the New York Academy of Medicine*, 98(Suppl 1), pp. 15–30. doi: 10.1007/s11524-021-00557-8.

Nowak, D. A. and Mulligan, K. (2021) 'Social prescribing: A call to action', *Canadian Family Physician Medecin de Famille Canadien*, 67(2), pp. 88–91. doi:10.46747/cfp.670288.

Sewdas, R. et al. (2019) 'Poor health, physical workload and occupational social class as determinants of health-related job loss: Results from a prospective cohort study in the UK', *BMJ Open*, 9(7), p. e026423. doi:10.1136/bmjopen-2018-026423.

White, A. et al. (2018) 'Social determinants of male health: A case study of Leeds, UK', *BMC Public Health*, 18(1), p. 160. doi:10.1186/s12889-018-5076-7.

Wildman, J. M. et al. (2019) 'Service-users' perspectives of link worker social prescribing: A qualitative follow-up study,' *BMC Public Health*, 19(1), p. 98. doi:10.1186/s12889-018-6349-x.

CHAPTER 23

The Biopsychosocial Model

The biopsychosocial model has been the main approach of several health care professions including occupational therapy, social work, physiotherapy, nursing, counselling and psychiatry (Frazier, 2020) since the late 20th century. The biopsychosocial model originated in the 1960s after the prevailing model within the medical community was the biomedical model and was officially attributed to Engel in 1977 (Engel, 1981). The key reason that a new model for healthcare was needed was that the biomedical model focussed on illness and disease and did not consider the whole person (Engel, 1981). A new perspective was needed because only considering the physical side of health and wellbeing is reductive and doesn't help to advance our understanding of the underlying causes of poor health or wellbeing (Frazier, 2020). Although it was originally published in 1977, the biopsychosocial model was only formally adopted and promoted by The World Health Organisation (WHO) in 2002 (Edwards, 2022). Engel's biopsychosocial model proposed that health is better understood through interconnected systems, those being; biological which predominantly focusses on disease and illness, psychological which is related to your thoughts, feelings and emotions and sociological being the context of a person's life (Keady et al., 2013). The 'social' aspect of the biopsychosocial model can relate not only to an individual's immediate social support but can also include their socioeconomic status and situation, where they live, their religion or the political system they are subject to (Frazier, 2020). The biopsychosocial model also helps us to understand the underlying determinants of health (Van de Velde et al., 2016). Psychological or social factors may not directly cause a health issue, but they are important factors in the treatment and recovery of all health issues (Frazier, 2020), and this can be due to the person's understanding of any illness they may have, motivation to engage with treatment interventions or ability to make lifestyle changes that could improve their health. Ultimately, the biopsychosocial model encompasses a whole person approach that has had a significant impact on all aspects of health and social care since its inception (Frazier, 2020).

In the field of mental health, we now understand that mental health issues and illnesses are impacted by all aspects of the biopsychosocial model (Chen et al., 2023). Dementia is a clear example of how the biopsychosocial model can be used to understand a condition

Thriving in Mental Health Nursing, First Edition. Laura Duncan.
© 2025 John Wiley & Sons Ltd. Published 2025 by John Wiley & Sons Ltd.

(Keady et al., 2013) as there are biological changes in the brain that impact memory; there are significant psychological considerations due to the confusion that can be experienced and an individual with dementia's social context is important as support from family and carer's can be crucial to enhancing wellbeing. In the field of child psychotherapy, where a psychological perspective has been the prevailing model historically, the role of the environment and biological considerations such as genetic predispositions to certain mental health conditions have become of increasing importance (Edwards, 2022), leading to greater adoption of the biopsychosocial model within the psychotherapy community. The impact of Adverse Childhood Experiences (ACEs) is a good example of a biopsychosocial understanding of the impact of psychological and social stressors on health (Frazier, 2020) as we now see crucial links between an individual experiencing multiple ACEs having a higher likelihood of developing mental and physical health issues in adulthood. Another important perspective for the biopsychosocial model is that of ageing well, and the biopsychosocial model helps to consider subjective wellbeing rather than just the consideration of disease or disability meaning that an individual can't 'age well', which is obviously not the case (Kanning and Schlicht, 2008).

In summary, for a biopsychosocial approach, the clinician must take both the person and their illness into account (Van de Velde et al., 2016) and using the biopsychosocial approach means that you will ultimately be delivering holistic and evidence-based care (Keady et al., 2013).

To understand the impact of biopsychosocial factors and how the interplay can affect and impact individuals, we will use a case study focussing on an individual with a diagnosis of schizophrenia to explore these concepts from a 'real world' perspective.

Schizophrenia Case Study

Sam is a 28-year-old male with a diagnosis of schizophrenia. He has had four admissions to inpatient mental health units since he was 23 and experienced his first episode of psychosis. Sam's mother and maternal aunt also have diagnoses of schizophrenia, and his sister has experienced a psychotic episode also during her 20s. Following his first three admissions, when he was discharged, he returned to the family home where he lives with his father, mother and sister. After his fourth admission, he moved to a supported accommodation facility. Due to her mental health issues, his mother has had frequent inpatient admissions and has been unable to work and his father is employed as a bus driver. The family have always struggled financially, and Sam recalls his parents frequently skipping meals, so he and his sister could eat. There were often arguments between Sam's parents that he remembers finding very frightening as they would frequently slam doors and his mother had occasionally thrown items such as plates and bowls at his father. Sam remembers his mum 'disappearing' for long periods of time, and when he would ask his father where she was and why she had gone away, his father would tell Sam and his sister that she was on holiday. Sam now realises that this must have been when his mother was receiving inpatient care and he finds it very difficult to talk about as he remembers feeling that his mother must not love him if she could leave for such long periods. Sam is also angry that his dad didn't tell him the truth as he could have visited his mum if he had known that she was in hospital. Sam remembers struggling in school and left without any formal qualifications. He worked in a supermarket and reported that he enjoyed his job as he got on well with his colleagues, but after his first episode of psychosis and being admitted to hospital for 6 weeks, he felt unable to return to work as he was embarrassed to explain why he had been absent for so long and he had received letters, whilst he was in hospital advising him that he was fired due to not showing up for his shifts.

After Sam had been discharged to his family home, his symptoms of psychosis were well managed and Sam was relieved to not be hearing voices anymore as he found them very upsetting and distressing. Sam's mother would tell him that there was nothing wrong with him or them and that he'd been given medication so that the government could control him. His sister had remained on medication for 2 years after her episode of psychosis and had not experienced any relapses after her medication was reduced and stopped. Sam's mother told him that his sister had foiled the government's plan and because she didn't need medication, neither did her or Sam. Sam initially didn't listen to his mum and continued taking his medication, but he did experience side effects of tiredness and lethargy so after several months, would start to think his mother was right and that he should stop taking his medication. This would then lead to Sam starting to hear the voices again which would affect his behaviour over time, and he would ultimately be re-admitted to hospital.

During his most recent admission, Sam told his care team what his mother would say to him and that she would encourage him to stop taking his medication, but that he hated the voices so much, he never wanted to experience them again; however, he found it difficult not to listen to his mother. This was when the team started exploring other accommodation options with Sam, and initially, he didn't want to leave the family home, but he ultimately understood that it was probably the best way for him to stay well and not experience the voices again. Sam also asked if there was a way he could not need to think about medication every day, so the team suggested he start a depot antipsychotic medication instead of taking tablets. Sam was relieved that there was an option that meant he wouldn't be tempted to stop taking the medication, so this was agreed as the best way forward.

Sam found living in the supported accommodation difficult and lonely. He had never lived alone and missed his family. He would visit his family most days, but he still found it challenging. He didn't speak to the other people living in the accommodation much and found most people weren't around much anyway. He found the staff to be nice, but they weren't there all the time. Sam had also never learned how to cook, so most of the time he just ate toast with jam. He told one of the staff this and that he missed his parents' cooking and having proper meals and so they said they would ask an Occupational Therapist (OT) to help him. Sam was thrilled when the OT showed him how to make basic meals, and they even found him cooking classes that he could attend. Sam loved the cooking classes and became more and more confident cooking and even began baking for the staff and other residents which helped him to make friends and feel less lonely at his accommodation.

From Sam's case study:

- What are the biological considerations for Sam?
- What are his psychological considerations?
- What are his social considerations?

Biological

There are several different biological considerations for Sam. First, we can see that there is a strong family history of schizophrenia and psychosis in Sam's family and this is evidence that Sam may have had a genetic predisposition to developing schizophrenia. Sam also needs to take medication for him to stay well, and this is clear from the fact that he has relapsed several times when he has stopped taking his medication. With medication, we also need to consider the physiological impact of this including side effects (such as lethargy and tiredness) but also long-term antipsychotic use and its impact on the cardiovascular system in particular. Due to this, Sam's physical health should be monitored regularly by his General Practitioner (GP) and care team to ensure he is staying physically healthy. Sam was also not eating well when he initially moved to the supported accommodation and having such a restricted diet of only eating toast and jam in the long term, could cause very significant physical health issues from him ultimately becoming malnourished.

Psychological

The psychological considerations for Sam are very important. Primarily, he is experiencing psychosis which is a psychological phenomenon within itself. Sam is also experiencing significant distress from the symptoms he experiences, and this will have a strong impact on his mood. Sam has also experienced several ACEs as he grew up in poverty, had a parent that experienced mental illness who was hospitalised multiple times and witnessed heated arguments throughout his childhood. These will have a significant impact on Sam's psychological wellbeing, and he experiences feelings of abandonment and anger towards his father from his childhood. Sam also experienced loneliness and isolation when first living in the supported accommodation which would further impact his mood. Due to these psychological considerations and their impact on Sam, he would benefit from talking therapies to help him process and move forward from the negative feelings he experiences in relation to his childhood and the distress from hearing voices in particular.

Social

Sam's social circumstances are complex, and he had difficulties at school and then felt unable to return to work he had previously enjoyed with his work opportunities being very limited from receiving no formal qualifications. There are difficult family dynamics, particularly in relation to his mother who encourages him to stop taking medication due to her own experiences of psychosis and symptoms of paranoia. Sam has limited positive support in his life due to the social issues within his family and has experienced financial difficulties and poverty throughout his childhood. Sam's social issues also include his inability to cook when he first moves to supported accommodation as he was never taught and didn't know where to start. OT intervention is crucial in these situations as being able to eat a balanced diet and knowing how to do that is key in living a healthy lifestyle.

From this case study, it is clear how the biopsychosocial model helps us to understand individuals from a holistic perspective and the importance of acknowledging and supporting individuals in each domain. This will ensure they receive appropriate support and care from different professionals to live their lives in the healthiest way possible to maintain their wellbeing not just physically but socially and psychologically as well.

References

Chen, L.H. et al. (2023) 'Editorial: The bio-psycho-social approach to understanding mental disorders', *Frontiers in Psychology*, 14. doi:10.3389/fpsyg.2023.1225433.

Edwards, J. (2022) 'A response piece to Ricky Emanuel's (2021) "Changing minds and evolving views: A bio-psycho-social model of the impact of trauma and its implications for clinical work" published in Issue 47.3 of this Journal', *Journal of Child Psychotherapy*, 48(2), pp. 303–307. doi:10.1080/0075417x.2022.2086900.

Engel, G.L. (1981) 'The clinical application of the biopsychosocial model', *The Journal of Medicine and Philosophy*, 6(2), pp. 101–124. doi:10.1093/jmp/6.2.101.

Frazier, L.D. (2020) 'The past, present, and future of the biopsychosocial model: A review of The Biopsychosocial Model of Health and Disease: New philosophical and scientific developments by Derek Bolton and Grant Gillett', *New Ideas in Psychology*, 57(100755), p. 100755. doi:10.1016/j.newideapsych.2019.100755.

Kanning, M. and Schlicht, W. (2008) 'A bio-psycho-social model of successful aging as shown through the variable "physical activity"', *European Review of Aging and Physical Activity: Official Journal of the European Group for Research into Elderly and Physical Activity*, 5(2), pp. 79–87. doi:10.1007/s11556-008-0035-4.

Keady, J. et al. (2013) 'Introducing the bio-psycho-social-physical model of dementia through a collective case study design', *Journal of Clinical Nursing*, 22(19–20), pp. 2768–2777. doi:10.1111/j.1365-2702.2012.04292.x.

Van de Velde, D. et al. (2016) 'How competent are healthcare professionals in working according to a bio-psycho-social model in healthcare? The current status and validation of a scale', *PLoS One*, 11(10), p. e0164018. doi:10.1371/journal.pone.0164018.

CHAPTER 24

The Stress Vulnerability Model

The stress vulnerability model by Zubin and Spring (1977) has become one of the most accepted models to explain why some individuals develop mental health issues and others do not. The model has been known as 'The Stress Vulnerability Model', 'The Stress-Diathesis Model', 'The Vulnerability Model' and 'The Vulnerability Stress Model' (Demke, 2022) in the literature but will be referred to as 'The Stress Vulnerability Model' throughout. Zubin and Spring (1977) developed the stress vulnerability model after finding that pre-existing models didn't provide a coherent or clear understanding of all of the interlinking factors that can lead to the development of schizophrenia specifically. The stress vulnerability model proposes that individuals may have a genetic predisposition to mental health conditions such as schizophrenia, but it is 'stressors' or 'protective factors' that impact whether an individual develops the condition or symptoms (Goldstein, 1990).

The stress vulnerability model was adapted to include all mental health issues rather than just being relevant to schizophrenia (Demke, 2022) and has now also been used to understand addictive behaviour with stressors such as being exposed to substance use increasing someone's likelihood of relapse of drug and/or alcohol use (Anderson, Ramo and Brown, 2006). Within the model, vulnerabilities were defined as those that are 'inborn' such as genetic factors and 'acquired' that can include complications during birth and delivery, trauma and social experiences (Zubin and Spring, 1977). The key premise of the model (shown below) is that those with high vulnerability are likely to develop symptoms at some point in their life whereas those with low vulnerability would ultimately need to experience a 'catastrophic' event to trigger a psychotic episode (Zubin and Spring, 1977) or other mental health conditions. Stressors such as bereavement, trauma or divorce have a significant impact on an individual's life, and they can play a significant role in the development of illness, both physical and psychological (Zubin and Spring, 1977).

Chapter 24 The Stress Vulnerability Model

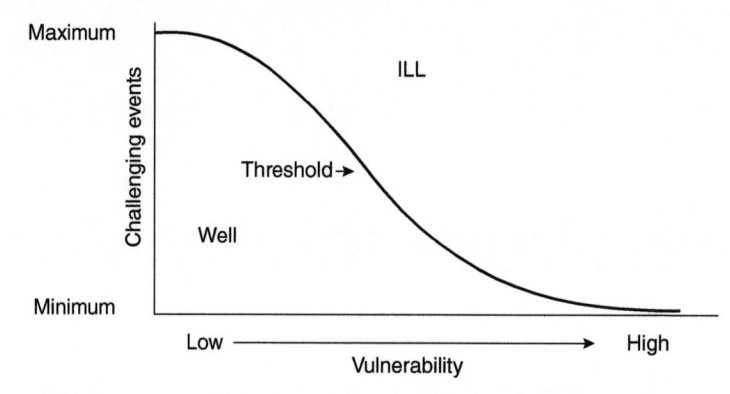

Figure: Stress Vulnerability Model showing Challenging events (Minimum to Maximum) on the y-axis and Vulnerability (Low to High) on the x-axis, with a threshold curve separating "Well" (below) from "ILL" (above) regions.

Source: Zubin et al. (1977)/with permission of American Psychological Association.

In relation to the figure above, stressful life events that stay below the threshold (signified by the line on the chart) mean the individual will remain well despite any challenges but those events that push someone above the line will mean they are likely to develop mental health issues. Factors that could mitigate someone's vulnerability would include their general personality traits, coping abilities and whether they have a good social network to 'cushion' the impact of any stressful life events (Nicholson and Neufield, 1992). General coping ability has been found to be a significant factor in mitigating the impact of life stressors (Anderson, Ramo and Brown, 2006) which highlights the importance of fostering healthy coping mechanisms before any stressful life events may occur. It has also been found that as we get older, our abilities to cope with stressors tends to increase (Charles, 2010), and this may be due to general increases in resilience as we grow older as well as stronger and more developed social networks. Zubin and Spring (1977) used an analogy of a string with a load attached, the string may be unaffected by the load, it may stretch and return to its usual length when the load is removed or the string may break. I find the string analogy to be a helpful visual representation of the model; some string may be able to withstand a heavy load, whereas another string may snap, but string can be tied back together and the repair may actually make the string stronger. There is a critique of the stress vulnerability model in that it actually reinforces the medical model approach and that individuals are inherently 'deficient' in some aspects if they have a high vulnerability to mental health issues (Demke, 2022); however, I would argue the opposite that it actually aligns much more closely with the biopsychosocial model in that it factors in an individual's response to stress and protective factors such as good social support. There is a lot of supporting evidence of genetic predispositions to conditions such as schizophrenia, bipolar affective disorder and depression, but the stress vulnerability model highlights that these pre-dispositions do not necessarily mean a person will develop symptoms. If they have a happy, secure and stable life, then they are very unlikely to ever develop any mental health conditions, but with enough exposure to stress or trauma, anyone could develop a mental health issue which is much more focussed on the psychological and social aspects of mental health.

Case Study

Siruti was born to two parents who both worked full time as estate agents. They had two other children and were able to be flexible with their work schedules, so they could attend school events and have one parent home with the children outside of school hours. Siruti enjoyed school and had lots of friends. She played football and was very active. Her parents had a stable and loving relationship, and Siruti remembers her childhood as being happy with lots of activities like going on bike rides and playing with her siblings. Siruti decided that she wanted to go to university to study English Literature as she loved reading. Her parents were very supportive and took her to see lots of different universities, so Siruti could decide where she wanted to study. She chose a university 4 hours away from home and was accepted. Siruti started university, and although she was nervous about being so far away from her family and friends, she was excited. She decided to join the university football society as soon as she arrived. She attended the try outs and wasn't selected for the team. Siruti was really upset by this as she loved playing football and thought it would be a good way to make friends. She started attending lectures and found that when she tried to start a conversation with people, they didn't seem to want to engage with her and would walk away. Siruti was also struggling to get on with the people in her halls. She found them very loud and brash; they would frequently be shouting and screaming during the night which she found very intimidating.

Siruti thought that this is probably how a lot of people felt during their first term at university and that she would start making friends soon. When she spoke to her family and friends at home, she found this made her very homesick and she didn't want them to worry, so she didn't tell them just how lonely she was feeling.

As the term progressed, her housemates all fell out with each other after several arguments had taken place and the atmosphere was very uncomfortable for Siruiti. She would generally just stay in her room when she wasn't in lectures. Siruti noticed that in her classes, it seemed that everyone else had made friends and were in groups. Whenever there was group work set, Siruti was too embarrassed to ask to join another group, so she wouldn't participate in the task. She failed an assignment as it was based on group work and when her lecturer asked her why she hadn't submitted her work, she told them she had been ill rather than explaining how difficult she was finding it.

Siruti went home for the Christmas break, and as the first person in her family to go to university, her parents and siblings asked lots of questions about how much fun she must be having and how many friends she must have made. Siruti lied and told her family that she was loving university life and couldn't wait to go back. The day she returned in January, Siruti went to her room and cried all night. She didn't know what to do, she didn't want to tell her family how bad it was, and although she desperately wanted to leave, she thought she would be a disappointment to her family if she did so.

Her next lecture was 2 days later, and Siruti hadn't left her room since she returned. She couldn't sleep as she was panicking about going to her next lecture, and when the time came to leave, she experienced her first panic attack, so she didn't go. Siruti then stopped attending lectures all together and only left her room to go to the shop downstairs to get food. Every time Siruti thought about seeing her housemates or going to a lecture, she just felt overwhelmed by panic. She could barely face going to the shop and so stopped eating regularly.

Siruti felt trapped and didn't know what she could do to improve the situation. Her mood became worse and worse and she began to have thoughts of ending her life. Siruti decided she would take an overdose and thought she would feel braver if she was drunk first, so she began drinking vodka.

Siruti normally did not drink alcohol and so she became drunk very quickly. She was crying loudly, and one of her housemates heard and knocked on her door. Siruti didn't answer the door, but they were worried and so walked in to find Siruti sat on the floor very distressed. She had several packs of paracetamol but had not taken any yet. The housemate was shocked and asked Siruti what was wrong and she told them that she wanted to die. They called the university porters for their accommodation for help, and a counsellor from the wellbeing service came to see Siruti straight away.

They talked to Siruti and gave her water; when she had sobered up, she was still very distressed, so they asked Siruti if it was ok to call her parents and let them know what was happening. Siruti agreed, and after hearing how distressed Siruti was, her parents immediately drove to her university to take her home.

Siruti withdrew from university, and her parents helped her to start counselling. She was diagnosed with anxiety and depression. Siruti started to feel better after a few weeks and, after six months at home, felt like herself again. She decided that she did want to study English at university but enrolled at a university near her home, so she could continue to live with her parents. After receiving help and support, she was excited to start a new chapter and found her second university experience to be much more enjoyable. She joined the football society and made lots of friends on her course. In her second year, she decided to live with friends rather than at home and enjoyed the rest of her degree.

As we can see in this case study, there was no indication of Siruti having a 'high vulnerability' to any mental health conditions; there is no known family history, for example, so we can consider her to have been 'low vulnerability'. Siruti had a comfortable and supportive upbringing, so it was only when she felt isolated and alone that any signs of mental health issues began to show. As we can see in this case study, Siruti's string could only hold so much weight. As someone who had a strong family support system, it was particularly challenging for her to feel so isolated and alone as she had never experienced this before. Her previous coping strategies of playing football weren't available to her, so she did not know how to manage the stressors she was experiencing. We could consider those coping strategies as things that will 'lighten the load' on the string and hold it up to minimise the impact of the weight exerted on the string. When we think about the stress vulnerability model, it is just as important to consider the impact of coping strategies and what happens if they are no longer available as it is to think about the impact of stress. 'Fixing the string' after it had broken in this scenario is when Siruti returned home to a supportive family and engaged with counselling. These factors helped Siruti to recover and 'repair the string' to the point she was able to return to university life with her key coping and protective factors in place, i.e. living at home.

The stress vulnerability model helps us to understand the impact of stress on us all; no one is immune to developing mental health issues if they are subjected to enough stress. One person may have the resilience and coping strategies to withstand pressures that others may not, and the model really highlights the importance of building resilience and healthy coping strategies for everyone. It also shows us that if someone does become unwell, that with the right help and support to reduce the stressors or impact of stressors, they can recover and 'fix the string'.

References

Anderson, K.G., Ramo, D.E. and Brown, S.A. (2006) 'Life stress, coping and comorbid youth: An examination of the stress-vulnerability model for substance relapse[dagger]', *Journal of Psychoactive Drugs*, 38(3), pp. 255–262.

Charles, S.T. (2010) 'Strength and vulnerability integration: A model of emotional well-being across adulthood,' *Psychological Bulletin*, 136(6), pp. 1068–1091. doi:10.1037/a0021232.

Demke, E. (2022) 'The vulnerability-stress-model-holding up the construct of the faulty individual in the light of challenges to the medical model of mental distress', *Frontiers in Sociology*, 7, p. 833987. doi:10.3389/fsoc.2022.833987.

Goldstein, M.J. (1990) 'Family relations as risk factors for the onset and course of schizophrenia', *Risk and Protective Factors in the Development of Psychopathology*. Cambridge University Press, pp. 408–423.

Nicholson, I.R. and Neufeld, R.W.J. (1992) 'A dynamic vulnerability perspective on stress and schizophrenia', *The American Journal of Orthopsychiatry*, 62(1), pp. 117–130. doi:10.1037/h0079307.

Zubin, J. and Spring, B. (1977) 'Vulnerability: A new view of schizophrenia', *Journal of Abnormal Psychology*, 86(2), pp. 103–126. doi:10.1037/0021-843x.86.2.103.

CHAPTER 25

Accessing Support

As mental health professionals, we focus our time and energy on supporting others through difficult times, usually with little thought of our own wellbeing. Due to this, there are high rates of stress and burnout amongst mental health professionals, and this is linked to issues such as vicarious traumatisation (Edwards and Crisp, 2016). When we consider the rates of distress, trauma and abuse that mental health professionals can experience as a standard part of their role, it is clear that this could have a negative impact over time. This can manifest in different ways for different people, but first responders in particular are exposed to frequent traumatic events which can have a significant impact on their mental health with rates of post-traumatic stress disorder amongst first responders being similar to armed forces veterans (Jones, Agud and McSweeney, 2019). There are many factors that can increase stress levels for clinical staff and high stress rates in nurses are linked to depression with nurses experiencing almost double the rates of depression compared to other professions (Lee, Jeong and Yi, 2020). Common features of healthcare professionals' roles such as shift work and irregular working patterns can also negatively affect the wellbeing of clinicians (Patel, Swift and Digesu, 2021). Nurses are at increased risk of depression and suicide, and this is largely attributed to work-based stress but also experiencing physical health issues or chronic pain, previous mental health issues, substance misuse or bereavement can significantly increase the risk of experiencing suicidality (Barnes et al., 2022). When there are co-occurring issues both inside and outside of the workplace, this can have a significant impact on the wellbeing and mental health of professionals. There was a significant increase in nurses attempting to take their own lives during the Covid-19 pandemic (Allen, 2021), and this is likely linked to many nurses feeling additional stress and pressure throughout the pandemic in both their personal and professional lives. For nurses, depression is also linked to burnout, wanting to leave the profession, fatigue and difficulties sleeping (Lee, Jeong and Yi, 2020). The impact of depression can also negatively impact functioning including reduced concentration and so can also negatively affect patient care (Lee, Jeong and Yi, 2020). This highlights that stress, depression and burnout not only affect the individual but also their ability to perform their role effectively. The key message from this is that if you struggle to prioritise your wellbeing for

Thriving in Mental Health Nursing, First Edition. Laura Duncan.
© 2025 John Wiley & Sons Ltd. Published 2025 by John Wiley & Sons Ltd.

yourself, you should consider that helping yourself will also help others. It appears that those who have been practicing longer appear more reticent to seek help and support than those newer to the profession (Edwards and Crisp, 2016), but feeling that you should be immune to experiencing stress or mental health issues due to being an experienced practitioner is clearly not logical or accurate.

As all mental health professionals know, seeking help early is key to recovery (Lee, Jeong and Yi, 2020). It is important both personally and professionally that individuals can disclose when they are struggling and feel confident in seeking help (Edwards and Crisp, 2016). This can be very challenging, but we should be advocating for nurses to seek help to reduce the numbers 'suffering in silence' (Barnes et al., 2022) whether that is for ourselves or our colleagues. As with other groups, for mental health professionals, stigma is a key factor in not seeking help (Edwards and Crisp, 2016). Alongside fearing stigma and discrimination, many mental health professionals cite concerns about privacy and confidentiality being a barrier to seeking help (Edwards and Crisp, 2016). It is concerning that professionals fear that if they disclose that they are struggling with their own mental health, this information would not be kept confidential. As individuals, we should feel confident in expressing our needs for support and advocating for our team members as well, but organisations should be more proactive in recognising the prevalence and impact of depression on nurses and offer more to support nurses (Lee, Jeong and Yi, 2020). Workplace initiatives that are targeted at promoting help-seeking and reducing stigma would be beneficial (Patel, Swift and Digesu, 2021), but these appear to be infrequent across the health and social care sector. Ultimately, while protecting clients, we must also protect ourselves (Patel, Swift and Digesu, 2021). The key to protecting ourselves is accessing help and support whenever we may need it.

Activity

There may have been times when you have felt your own mental health or wellbeing was less than optimal. If you have already experienced this, take some time to consider what actions you took or support you received that may have helped you recover and move forward. Reflect on whether you sought support as early as you could have done, or did you 'suffer in silence'?

Take some time to consider the following questions:

- What do you think you can do to maintain your wellbeing?
- How do you maintain your work/life balance?
- What do you think could be your 'early warning signs' that your mental health is deteriorating?
- Who would you feel comfortable talking to?
- How would you feel about seeking professional help?
- What would you do if you felt a colleague was struggling with their mental health?
- What would you do if there had been a particularly difficult situation or incident in work?

Some of these questions may have been easier to answer than others, but it is important to consider what we would do if we or a colleague were having a difficult time. Below are some points to consider to maintain our own wellbeing as professionals but also tips for what to do if we feel that we are starting to experience issues or feel a colleague is:

- Try to maintain a good work/life balance. It is easy when we have a demanding role to prioritise that over our personal lives but make sure you are taking time to look after yourself, not just looking after others. This could be engaging in self-care activities, hobbies, seeing friends and family, etc., but also includes making sure you are eating well, drinking enough water and getting enough sleep and rest.
- Think about your network. If you have a bad day or are starting to feel burned out, plan who you would talk to first. This could be a friend or family member, but if you are experiencing stress, burnout or feel your mental health is deteriorating, you also need to speak to your team manager. That can be really challenging depending on your relationship with them, but it is important that your manager knows if you are struggling so that they can support you.
- Think about what you would advise if someone told you they were feeling how you have been. What would you suggest they do? Take your own advice!
- Take breaks and annual leave. We all know how difficult it can be to take breaks, leave on time or book leave, but it is so important to get adequate rest and have regular breaks from work. Try to spread your leave throughout the year, so you know when you have time off coming up. Don't agree to work extra shifts or cover short staffing issues all the time as it can be so difficult to say 'no' when we know how hard it is when there are poor staffing levels, but working too much is detrimental to not only our mental health but also our physical health.
- If you feel burned out, take a break. You may need to be off sick for a week if you act quickly, but if you continue pushing yourself to breaking point, then you may be off sick for a much longer period.
- Speak to your General Practitioner (GP). We sometimes think as mental health professionals we should be immune or able to treat ourselves when we are struggling with our mental health, but exactly as we would advise others, if you are experiencing anxiety or low mood, you need to speak to your GP.
- Seek therapy or counselling. It is ok if you are worried about being a patient in the same trust or area where you are a professional, you are allowed to have those boundaries and they should be supported. Speak to your GP or local counselling service about getting 'out of area' support or consider finding a private counsellor if you would prefer to keep your care completely separate. You can also contact your organisation's employee assistance programme who should be able to offer confidential support and counselling.
- Know you don't have to feel like this. Nursing is a high-stress job, but you don't need to personally suffer to be a good nurse. Most mental health professionals will struggle at one point in their career, and there is no shame in that. Seek help, support and take a break if you are not ok, the same as you would advise a colleague to if they told you they were feeling low or struggling with their mental health.
- Look out for your colleagues. If a colleague seems to be behaving differently or isn't their normal selves, check in on them. Let's normalise talking to our team when things are tough. Role model what you would like others to do for you if you weren't feeling or acting like yourself.
- Debrief and engage with reflective practice. Difficult or traumatic incidents can occur in mental health; we need to be accepting that this can affect us deeply as individuals and as a team. Giving everyone the time and space to express their thoughts and feelings in a supportive, caring environment following a difficult situation is vital and should be standard practice.

- If you feel that you can't keep yourself safe or are having thoughts of suicide, seek urgent help. You matter, you are important and you deserve support. Tell a friend, call a helpline, go to the Emergency Department (also known as Accident and Emergency or A&E) or call an ambulance. You won't always feel this way, so let others help you the way you help so many.

As mental health professionals, we frequently advise others that 'you can't pour from an empty cup', but do we always listen to our own advice? We can't be effective if we are struggling, so it is vital that we pay attention to our own needs and feelings before we focus on those of others. We can build positive cultures where all professionals feel comfortable and able to ask for help when they need it. If you can't do it for yourself, do it as a role model to others who may not have the confidence to reach out for help.

If you are struggling with your mental health or having thoughts of suicide, please seek help now. Contact your GP, employee assistance programme, your local crisis line or call Samaritans on 116 123.

References

Allen, D. (2021) 'Shame and stigma: Why nurses fear seeking help when they reach rock bottom', *Mental Health Practice*, 24(6), pp. 6–8. doi:10.7748/mhp.24.6.6.s2.

Barnes, A. et al. (2022) 'Entangled: A mixed method analysis of nurses with mental health problems who die by suicide', *Nursing Inquiry*, 30(2). doi:10.1111/nin.12537.

Edwards, J.L. and Crisp, D.A. (2016) 'Seeking help for psychological distress: Barriers for mental health professionals', *Australian Journal of Psychology*, 69(3), pp. 218–225. doi:10.1111/ajpy.12146.

Jones, S., Agud, K. and McSweeney, J. (2019) 'Barriers and facilitators to seeking mental health care among first responders: "Removing the Darkness"', *Journal of the American Psychiatric Nurses Association*, 26(1), p. 107839031987199. doi:10.1177/1078390319871997.

Lee, E., Jeong, Y.M. and Yi, S.J. (2020) 'Nurses' attitudes toward psychiatric help for depression: The serial mediation effect of self-stigma and depression on public stigma and attitudes toward psychiatric help. *International Journal of Environmental Research and Public Health*, 17(14), p. 5073. doi:10.3390/ijerph17145073.

Patel, M., Swift, S. and Digesu, A. (2021) 'Mental health among clinicians: What do we know and what can we do?', *International Urogynecology Journal*, 32(5). doi:10.1007/s00192-021-04805-y.

CHAPTER 26

Final Thoughts

Mental health nursing is a complex and challenging profession. Depending on the nature of the work we do, we will experience trauma, distress and conflict on an almost daily basis. How to work effectively with clients who are experiencing distress has been explored, but the key theme throughout is how to be reflective practitioners that recognise the impact the work may have on us and what to do about it. We work in teams generally speaking, so ensuring that we support ourselves and our colleagues leads to improved wellbeing and satisfaction. As discussed, many nurses consider leaving the profession and there can be many multifaceted reasons for this. Most commonly though, this will be due to stress, burnout or poor job satisfaction. If we can recognise the emotional impact of the work and be proactive in addressing that through self-care and seeking support, then stress levels and burnout will be reduced. If someone is not enjoying their role, considering their professional development and the style of work they would prefer is an important consideration.

Leadership has been considered extensively with an emphasis on compassionate leadership and supporting others. With effective and kind leadership, we can see whole teams perform better but also thrive rather than simply survive. There is a general feeling that student nurses and early-career nurses are not well supported; there are limitless potential reasons for this, both individual or organisational, but we must focus on being positive role models and leaders for the next generation of nurses. It can be challenging, but we need to show others the nurse we want them to be.

There are undoubtedly significant challenges ahead for the profession and if we are to be the best nurses we can be and maintain our wellbeing, we need to support one another practically and proactively. Be the leader you wanted to see, use your voice to improve services for clients and staff and care for yourself the way you care for others.

Thriving in Mental Health Nursing, First Edition. Laura Duncan.
© 2025 John Wiley & Sons Ltd. Published 2025 by John Wiley & Sons Ltd.

INDEX

A
ableism, 51
accessing support
   activity, 182–184
   Covid-19 pandemic, 181
   depression, 181
   suffering in silence, 182
   vicarious traumatisation, 181
ACEs *see* adverse childhood experiences (ACEs)
active listening skills, 26
Activities of Daily Living assessments, 42
adverse childhood experiences (ACEs), 33, 34, 52, 70, 170
alleviating suffering, 83
antisemitism, 52
authoritative leaders, 138
autism spectrum disorder (ASD), 70, 71

B
biopsychosocial model, 1
   age well, 170
   case study
      biological, 171–172
      psychological, 172
      schizophrenia, 170–171
      social, 172
   dementia, 169–170
   Engel's biopsychosocial model, 169
   social aspect, 169
bipolar affective disorder, 116–117
burnout
   career, 103
   case study, 105–107
   definition, 101
   emotional and physical symptoms, 101
   moderate–severe levels of, 103
   negative impact, work, 104–105
   severity, pervasiveness and consequence of, 101
   signs of, 101
   workload, 104

C
Child and Adolescent Mental Health Services (CAMHS), 21, 50, 92
chronic obstructive pulmonary Disease (COPD), 35, 69
chronic stress, 96
clinical supervision, 147, 148
CLW *see* Community Link Worker (CLW)
coercive practices, 123–124
communication
   autistic spectrum disorder, 26
   case study, 28–31
   definition, 25
   felt unheard, 27–28
   good teamwork, 25
   hearing or vision loss, 26
   person-centred, 25
   positive caring relationships, 25
   reflection, 27
   role-modelling, 27
   role-play, 27
   schizophrenia, 25
   therapeutic relationships with clients, 25
   written, 25
Community Link Worker (CLW), 166, 167
compassion
   activity, 85–86
   case study, 86–88
   definition, 83
   empathy and sympathy, 83
   Francis Report (2013), 84
   interpersonal and listening skills, 85

Thriving in Mental Health Nursing, First Edition. Laura Duncan.
© 2025 John Wiley & Sons Ltd. Published 2025 by John Wiley & Sons Ltd.

compassionate leadership, 83, 137, 139–140
compassion fatigue, 34–36, 83, 85–86
complexity
  activity, 71–72
  ASD, 70, 71
  case study, 72–73
  comorbidity, 69
  definition, 69
  environmental or behavioural issues, 69
  IDD, 70
conflict
  activity, 76–79
  case study, 78–81
  de-escalation techniques, 76
  early warning signs, 76
  positive therapeutic relationships, 75
  PRN, 75
  restrictive practices, 75
COPD *see* chronic obstructive pulmonary Disease (COPD)
coronavirus disease 2019 (COVID-19) pandemic, 7, 95, 101, 159, 161, 181
courtesy stigma, 109, 110–111
COVID-19 pandemic *see* coronavirus disease 2019 (COVID-19) pandemic
cultural competence, 49, 55, 56

D

de-escalation techniques, 76
delegative leaders, 138, 139
dementia, 71, 169–170
Department of Health (1983), 122–124
disability, 51
discrimination, 52–53
diversity and inclusivity
  activity, 56–57
  definition, 49
  ethical practice, 49
  Protected Characteristics, 50
    age, 50
    disability, 51
    gender reassignment, 53
    marriage and civil partnership, 50
    pregnancy and maternity, 50
    racism, 51
    religion, 52–53
    sex, 53–54
    sexual orientation, 54–55
Driscoll's Model of Reflection, 6–8

E

effective listening, 26
emotional intelligence
  activity, 20–21
  case study, 21–23
  definition, 19
  high levels of, 19
  impact of, 20
  self-awareness, 19
  training, 20
Engel's biopsychosocial model, 169
Equality Act (2010), 50
ethical practice
  autonomy, 121
  beneficence, 122
  case study, 125–126
  character and values, 123
  coercive practices, 123–124
  justice, 122
  moral sensitivity, 123
  non-maleficence, 122
  patient outcome, 126
  utilitarianism, 122

F

Forensic Mental Health services, 41
formative supervision, 148, 149
Francis Report (2013), 84

G

gender discrimination, 53–54
Gibbs' reflective cycle, 3–4
Gibbs' reflective model, 4–6

H

Health and Social Care, 129
hearing or vision loss, 26
homelessness, 159
hope
  acute or inpatient services, 89
  case study, 89–93
  definition, 89
hypervigilance, 34

I

individual lifestyle factors, 161
informal reflective principles, 7–8
intellectual and/or developmental disorders (IDDs), 69, 70

intentional misgendering, 55
Islamophobia, 52

J
job application, 155–156
job interview, 156–158

K
King's fund (1993), 160

L
leadership, 185
  activity, 144–145
  authoritative, 138
  case studies, 140–143
  compassionate, 137, 139–140
  delegative, 138, 139
  participative, 138, 139
  positive, 137
  quality, 137
  servant, 139
  transactional, 138
  transformational, 138, 139
LGBTQ+, 54–55
listening
  active listening skills, 26
  activity, 27–28
  case study, 28–31
  definition, 26
  effective, 26
  reflection, 27
  role-modelling, 27
  role-play, 27
  therapeutic communication skills, 26
  therapeutic interactions, 26
Living and Working Conditions, 161

M
macro-aggressions, 52
managerial supervision, 147
marriage and civil partnership, 50
MDT *see* multidisciplinary team (MDT)
Mental Health Act (1983), 63, 78, 110, 121
Mental Health professionals, 1
micro-aggressions, 52
Mid-Staffordshire NHS Foundation Trust, 84
moral distress, 12
moral sensitivity, 123
multidisciplinary team (MDT), 43, 125, 129, 130

N
National Health Service's (NHS), 114–115
  burnout, 101
  5 Steps to Well-being
    Be physically active, 98
    Connect with other people, 97–98
    Give to others, 98–99
    Learn new skills, 98
    Pay attention to the present moment, 99
  healthcare services case study, 163, 164
  '6 C's', 84
National Institute of Clinical Health and Excellence 2015 (NICE), 77
NHS *see* National Health Service's (NHS)
normative supervision, 148, 149
Nursing and Midwifery Council (NMC), 3, 123, 148

O
obsessive compulsive disorder (OCD), 115–116
Office for National Statistics 2021 (ONS), 53

P
participative leadership, 138, 139
paternalistic approaches, 122
perceived discrimination, 50
person-centred communication, 25
physical health presenteeism, 13
PICU *see* psychiatric intensive care unit (PICU)
positive team working, 129
post-traumatic stress disorder (PTSD) symptoms, 34, 35
presenteeism, 13
primary stressor, 51
Proctor's model of clinical supervision
  formative supervision, 148, 149
  normative supervision, 148, 149
  restorative supervision, 148, 149
professional development
  activity
    career, 154
    job application, 155–156
    job interview, 156–158
    portfolio, 155
  definition, 153
Pro Re Nata (PRN), 75
Protected Characteristics, 50
  age, 50
  disability, 51
  gender reassignment, 53
  marriage and civil partnership, 50

Protected Characteristics
  pregnancy and maternity, 50
  racism, 51–52
  religion, 52–53
  sex, 53–54
  sexual orientation, 54–55
provider-based stigma, 109, 111
psychiatric intensive care unit (PICU), 72, 91, 131, 143, 144
psychological trauma, 33
public stigma, 109, 110

Q
quality leadership, 137

R
racism, 51–52
Rainbow Model, The, 160
rapid cycling bipolar, 116
Recovery Star, 92, 93
reflection
  activity, 4, 8–9
  Driscoll's Model of Reflection, 6–7
  Gibbs' reflective cycle, 3–4
  Gibbs' reflective model, 4–6
  informal reflective principles, 7–8
  NMC standards, 3
reflective practitioner, 3, 4, 8, 97, 185
regular supervision, 148
religious discrimination, 52–53
resilience
  activity, 14–15
  clinical practice, 15–17
  critical aspects of, 14
  definition, 11, 12
  fundamental cultural and organisational issue, 13
  increasing our personal, 13
  presenteeism, 13
  stress and stressors, 11
  team member, 13
restorative supervision, 148, 149
risk
  assessment, 42–43
  case study, 43–47
  definition, 41
  maintaining safety and managing, 41
  MDT, 43
  positive risk-taking, 43
risk aversion, 42
role-modelling, 27
role-play, 27
Royal College of Nurses (RCN), 148

S
schizophrenia, 25, 72, 89, 114, 116, 170–171, 175, 176
secondary traumatic stress, 34, 35
self-awareness, 19
self-care, 2
self-care and well-being
  activities
    Be physically active, 98
    Connect with other people, 97–98
    Give to others, 98–99
    Learn new skills, 98
    Pay attention to the present moment, 99
  chronic stress, 96
  COVID-19 pandemic, 95
  examples of, 96
self-stigma, 111–115
servant leadership, 139
'6 C's' (care, compassion, competence, courage, communication and commitment), 84
Social and Community Networks, 161
social determinants of health
  case study
    agriculture and food production, 161
    education, 161
    healthcare services, 163–164
    housing, 164–166
    social prescribing, 166–167
    unemployment, 162–163
    water and sanitation, 163
    work environment, 162
  Covid-19 pandemic, 159
  definition, 159
  homelessness, 159
  individual lifestyle factors, 161
  life expectancy gap, 159
  Living and Working Conditions, 161
  Social and Community Networks, 161
Social Readjustment Rating Scale, 11
stigma and discrimination, 51
  asylums, 117
  being kind, 118
  bipolar, 116–117
  case study
    courtesy stigma, 110–111
    provider-based stigma, 111
    public stigma, 110
    self-stigma, 111–115
    structural stigma, 110
  challenge others, 118
  OCD, 115–116
  schizophrenia, 116
Stress-Diathesis Model, The, 175

stressful occupation, 12
stress vulnerability model, 1, 11
   bipolar affective disorder, 176
   case study, 177–178
   catastrophic, 175
   depression, 176
   schizophrenia, 175
structural stigma, 109, 110
supervision skills
   benefits of, 147
   case study, 150–152
   clinical, 147, 148
   managerial, 147
   Proctor's model, 148–149
   reflective activity, 150
   regular supervision, 148

T

team working
   case study
      avoiding, 133–134
      compromising, 132
      dominating, 132–133
      integrating, 131–132
      obliging, 134–135
   challenges, 129
   communication, 130
   conflict, 130–131
   core benefit of, 129
   MDT, 129, 130
   positive feedback, 130
   positive team working, 129
   training, 130
therapeutic communication skills, 26
therapeutic relationships
   core traits of, 62
   definition, 61
   developing and maintaining, 62
   development, 63–65
   development or continuation, 63
   ending stages, 66
   maintenance, 65–66
   power imbalance, 63
   quality of, 62
Time off in lieu (TOIL), 104
transactional leadership, 138, 139
Trans community, 55
transformational leadership, 138
trauma
   ACE, 33, 34
   case study, 36–39
   definition, 33
   effects of, 34
   hypervigilance, 34
   impacts of, 35
   research, 35
   TIC, 36
   vicarious traumatisation, 35
trauma-informed care (TIC), 36

U

unconscious bias, 56
utilitarianism, 122

V

vicarious traumatisation, 35, 36, 181
virtue ethics, 123
vulnerability model, 175

W

workaholic, 35
working
   with risk
      assessment, 42–43
      case study, 43–47
      definition, 41
      maintaining safety and managing, 41
      MDT, 43
      positive risk-taking, 43
   in teams
      case study, 131–135
      challenges, 129
      communication, 130
      conflict, 130–131
      core benefit of, 129
      MDT, 129, 130
      positive feedback, 130
      positive team working, 129
      training, 130
   with trauma
      ACE, 33, 34
      case study, 36–39
      definition, 33
      effects of, 34
      hypervigilance, 34
      impacts of, 35
      research, 35
      TIC, 36
      vicarious traumatisation, 35
World Health Organisation (WHO), 160, 169
written communication, 25